The Hypothyroid Syndrome

By
Dr Peter Baratosy MBBS FACNEM

Dr Peter Baratosy is a registered Medical Doctor in Australia. He graduated from the University of Adelaide Medical School in 1978. He is a Fellow of the Australasian College of Nutritional and Environmental Medicine and is an accredited Medical Acupuncturist with the Medical Board of Australia.

Published by Dr Peter Baratosy 2023

Copyright Dr Peter Baratosy 2023

Cover Design: Nikola Boskovski

Editor: Karen Mace

ISBN - 978-0-6451053-3-9 (print version)

978-0-6451053-4-6 (eBook version)

I dedicate this book, as always, to my better half, Jenny, without whom I would not have been able to achieve writing this book. Thank you for your ongoing love, support, and encouragement.

This book is written for general information only. It is not intended for diagnosis or treatment.

The author, editor and publisher accept no responsibility for any adverse reaction caused by lack of consultation with a qualified doctor or practitioner, including responsibility for any personal decisions made by the reader in relation to his or her or any member of their family's self-diagnosis.

Table of Contents

PART 1

Chapter 1
Introduction

I am a clinician with a strong interest in thyroid disease. I started treating those who came to me with hypothyroid issues complaining that they were still not feeling well despite being treated. They came to me because I had developed a reputation for treating thyroid problems that others could not. Other doctors initially diagnosed these people with hypothyroidism, mainly Hashimoto's thyroiditis. They presented to their doctor with signs and symptoms of hypothyroidism, such as tiredness, weight gain, coldness, brain fog, constipation, and dry hair/dry skin, and were correctly diagnosed the conventional way with a blood test. Their thyroid stimulating hormone (TSH) was elevated, and they had a low thyroxine (T4) level.

So far so good! The diagnosis was correct. They were then started on the orthodox approved treatment, levothyroxine, a synthetic form of T4. Follow-up showed that their TSH had come down to normal and their T4 had come up to normal. However, and this is the big however, they were still *not* feeling well. They kept many of their hypothyroid symptoms, perhaps not as badly, *but* they were still not feeling as well as they thought they should be. They went back to their doctor, who basically told them that their thyroid test was normal, and therefore, their symptoms could not be because of their thyroid.

This explanation did not satisfy them. They talked with friends, some who were in the same situation, they searched the internet; they looked at various thyroid fora, and they concluded that they still could be hypothyroid. They went back multiple times to their doctor and complained. Because the blood test was "normal", the doctor still refused to accept that they still may be hypothyroid.

This made me realise there was a problem.

What were we missing?

After much research and thinking, I began to find solutions. I developed a reputation for successfully treating people like those described above. The secret of my success is that I look at the person from a wholistic point of view. I realised that treating hypothyroidism is not just replacing hormones. The other thing I discovered was that many of these people did not respond to levothyroxine (synthetic T4) alone. I only discovered later why this may be so, and this will be revealed later. I started treating people with added triiodothyronine (T3), which deviated from the orthodox viewpoint of thyroid treatment. The mainstream protocol basically stipulated that the **only** treatment for hypothyroidism was synthetic T4 (levothyroxine).

Why are the thyroid hormones called T4 and T3?

The T4 thyroid hormone is an inactive pro-hormone which has four iodine molecules attached while the T3, which is the active hormone, has three iodine molecules attached. In the process of activating the hormone, one iodine is removed from T4 to produce T3. This process requires an enzyme, and this occurs not in the blood stream but intracellularly. Every cell in the body must do this conversion otherwise the cell cannot function properly. Thyroid hormone will not work if it cannot be converted to the active form.

I also started using the natural form of thyroid hormone, the desiccated thyroid (DT). This consists of animal thyroid glands, mostly of porcine origin, that are dried, granulated, then put into capsules. This is the original form of hypothyroid treatment that originated at the end of the 1800s. In fact, the only treatment for hypothyroidism back then was animal thyroid replacement.

The combination of T3 and T4, or DT, worked better that synthetic T4 alone in these special situations.

DT contains not just T4, but T3 and other components of thyroid including T2 and T1, and a host of other hormones, substances known and possibly not known. It is a <u>complete</u> replacement – not just a <u>partial</u> replacement. Why replace only T4 when the thyroid secretes mainly T4 but also some T3?

This never make sense to me.

Since many hypothyroid people came to me with the same situation, I began to think that the synthetic T4 did not work at all. Let's look at this from another perspective–only those that didn't respond to T4 alone self-referred themselves to me–I only saw that select group. I later realised that T4 alone does work with many people, however, they generally do not come to see me.

There is a group, a subset of hypothyroid people, for whom the T4 alone did not produce a significant clinical result but the added T3, or the DT did.

What is different about these people?

> There is a subgroup of hypothyroid people who responded better to combination therapy than to monotherapy.

There were some people who were not interested in taking animal thyroids; this group included vegetarians and vegans. Jewish, and Muslim people mostly would not take the DT because it was from a pig, and there were some who just weren't keen on "eating" animal thyroids.

In these situations, I added a dose of T3 to their T4 replacement, which also produced dramatic improvements. I did not use the standard form of T3; I used a compounded product made up by compounding pharmacists, a slow-release form of T3, (SR T3). Be aware that commercial pharmaceutical companies do *not* make a slow-release form of T3.

I used the compounded slow-release form because it only needed to be taken once a day whereas the standard formulation has a quick action, a short half-life, which means that small frequent doses are needed every 3-4 hours.

The bottom line was that I treated this group with "combination therapy", i.e., T3 + T4. This includes DT as it contains T3 and T4 and others, and not "monotherapy" (T4 only), and they responded well.

My reputation for successfully treating hypothyroidism grew. I had people consulting me from all over Tasmania, and even some from interstate.

Dr Peter Baratosy MBBS FACNEM

The next group of people that came to me were those with normal blood tests despite having hypothyroid symptoms. Like the others I was seeing, these patients were told by their doctor that because the blood test was normal, they could not have thyroid disease. These people were still not well; they were suffering with typical hypothyroid symptoms. Their quality of life was poor; they could not function properly at work, at home, as a mother or father, as a wife or husband, as a person.

The following case study is a typical story.

A young lady consulted me after being referred by a friend. She gave a history of developing Graves' disease (autoimmune hyperthyroidism), and being treated with radioactive iodine, basically to kill off (nuke) her thyroid gland. Afterwards, as you would expect, she became progressively hypothyroid. She developed the typical symptoms of coldness, tiredness, weight gain, brain fog, poor thinking, and poor concentration. The endocrinologist started her on levothyroxine which she said did help a little, but she continued to be cold, lethargic, and tired, as well as gaining weight and most particularly suffering ongoing brain fog. The endocrinologist did blood tests which came back as normal and dismissed her. She went back repeatedly but to no avail.

14

Eventually, she lost her job because of her tiredness and inability to concentrate. After listening to her story when she consulted me, I was sure I knew what was going on; she was clinically hypothyroid but biochemically normal. A close look at her blood results showed that her TSH and T4 were normal. T3 levels were not done. I repeated the tests, and I also requested a T3 level; the result showed a very low normal T3. I added a dose of SR T3 to her existing levothyroxine, and after a short time of fine tuning her dose she improved greatly and is now back at work.

I treated these clinically hypothyroid, but biochemically normal, people with vitamins and minerals and herbs, as we shall discuss later, as well as thyroid replacement: I prescribed either levothyroxine, or levothyroxine with added SRT3, or DT, and they improved dramatically.

At this point, I started getting rumblings from the endocrinologists. "Why are you treating these people with thyroid replacement when they 'do not have thyroid disease'?" I tried to explain my thinking. They refused to listen. They accused me of over-diagnosing hypothyroidism. I responded by saying that they were under-diagnosing hypothyroidism.

The bottom line was that those who came to see me improved their quality of life by being supplemented with thyroid hormone. From a safety viewpoint, and to avoid possible over-replacement, I monitored them with regular blood checks and regular clinical follow up. Even though their blood tests were initially normal, adding extra thyroid hormone did not seem to cause them to become hyperthyroid (over-replaced). The dose was appropriate; enough to make them feel better, but not enough to over-replace them. At the same time, I also gave dietary advice, supplemented nutrients and herbs and tried to improve other aspects of their health.

Another controversy I have been involved in was with the "suppressed TSH" that some developed. To achieve good clinical outcomes, some people need a higher dose of replacement. In the orthodox paradigm, a suppressed TSH indicates hyperthyroidism, or an over-replacement of levothyroxine. However, if there are no symptoms of over-replacement and the levels of T3 and T4 are quite normal, how can they be over-replaced?

Some people need extra thyroid replacement to make them feel better/normal. Some accept TSH suppression to get an adequate dose to relieve their symptoms. So, is it better to focus on the person or the blood test?

I have received letters from endocrinologists expressing concern that a person's TSH was suppressed, which may lead to heart disease and osteoporosis.

However, the factor that leads to osteoporosis and heart disease is an elevated T3 and T4, not necessarily a suppressed TSH. I consistently monitor these people and even though the TSH is suppressed, the T3 and T4 levels are quite normal.

Some studies show that bone metabolism is related to TSH levels, and therefore if the TSH is low, this may then affect the bone. Abe et al. (2003) demonstrated that TSH receptors are found in bone cells, the osteoclasts, and the osteoblasts, and this leads to the idea that TSH could influence the bones. It is well accepted that hyperthyroidism can lead to osteoporosis due to the increased metabolic rate. This is because of the elevation of T3 and T4, not necessarily because of the suppression of TSH.

There have been many studies looking at this. The results are contradictory and inconclusive, as some studies show osteoporosis with suppressed TSH, and other studies do not.

Below are some of the studies that demonstrate both outcomes.

Garin, Arnold, Lee, Robbins, and Cappola (2014) showed no association between subclinical hypothyroidism or subclinical hyperthyroidism and hip fracture risk of bone mineral density (BMD) in older men and women.

Note: Subclinical hyperthyroidism is where there is a suppressed TSH but normal T3 and T4. Subclinical hypothyroidism is where there is an elevated TSH and normal T3 and T4.

Grant, McMurdo, Mole, Paterson, and Davies (1993) showed TSH suppression from TH replacement is not associated with osteoporosis.

The study by Papadimitriou, Papadimitriou, Papadopoulou, Nicolaidou, and Fretzayas (2007) showed no association between low TSH levels and osteoporosis in childhood. Poomthavorn, Mahachoklertwattana, Ongphiphadhanakul, Preeyasombat, and Rajatanavin (2005) also showed that exogenous subclinical hyperthyroidism has no effect on peak bone density in adolescents.

Current clinical practice recommends suppressive doses of thyroxine to suppress TSH for treatment of thyroid cancer after thyroidectomy.

Zhang, Xi, and Yan (2018) showed TSH suppression therapy had little effect on bone density in postmenopausal women being treated for differentiated thyroid cancer.

Fujiyama et al. (1995) demonstrated no acceleration of bone loss in postmenopausal women treated for thyroid cancer with suppressive doses of thyroxine. In a systematic overview of the literature, Quan, Pasieka, and Rorstad (2002) also came to the same conclusion, although, *"Findings for postmenopausal women remain unclear with two of the best controlled studies reporting opposing results."*

In another study, Marcocci, Golia, Bruno-Bossio, Vignali, and Pinchera (1994) showed no bone loss in premenopausal women with suppressive therapy. In a more recent study, Lee et al. (2014) also came to the same conclusion, even with supraphysiologically suppressed TSH.

Bauer, Nevitt, Ettinger, and Stone (1997) found no consistent evidence between low TSH levels and low BMD.

Bassett et al. (2007) showed that osteoporosis in hyperthyroidism is produced by thyroid hormone excess and not by TSH deficiency.

However, there are some studies that do show a relationship, although there may be confounding factors involved.

Blum et al. (2015) showed increased hip and other bone fractures particularly among those with TSH levels of less than 0.10 mIU/L and in those with endogenous subclinical hyperthyroidism.

Note that endogenous subclinical hyperthyroidism is caused by some internal disease, e.g., early Graves' disease, while levothyroxine replacement can cause exogenous subclinical hyperthyroidism.

Grimnes, Emaus, Joakimsen, Figenschau, and Jorde (2008) demonstrated lower bone density in men and women with a *"serum TSH consistent with hyperthyroidism"* than those with normal TSH.

Swathi, Haseena, and Saheb Shaik (2014) conclude *"The patients on long term treatment of drugs like levothyroxine, in spite of treating hypothyroidism there is a loss of bone mineral density although not with a higher fracture rate due to suppression of TSH levels."*

Svare et al. (2009) concluded that in women with self-reported hyperthyroidism, the prevalence of osteoporosis was higher in women with the lowest TSH levels. The question here is, Is this due to the low TSH, or to the "self-reported" hyperthyroidism?

Baqi et al. (2010) showed that TSH "normal" levels conceivably have a positive role in influencing bone density – irrespective of T4 levels.

Waring et al. (2013) determined *"We conclude that although neither TSH nor FT4 are associated with bone loss, lower serum TSH may be associated with an increased risk of hip fractures in older men."* Again, is this related to low TSH, or to ageing?

Mazziotti et al. (2005) determined that levothyroxine suppressive therapy, bone mass loss is more marked in postmenopausal women than in premenopausal women. However, we should mention that bone mass loss can be a part of post menopause.

Batrinos (2006) maintains that *".... it is the free thyroid hormones values in the serum that generate and reflect the thyroid metabolic state of the organism rather than the degree of TSH suppression."*

Bauer et al. (2004) concluded, *"the study did not demonstrate evidence that long term treatment of affectively ill patients with supraphysiological doses of L-T4 significantly accelerates loss of bone mineral...."* However, they do recommend caution as *one patient* of the group of 21 in the study did have BMD decline, so the researchers cautioned that *"regular assessment of BMD during longer-term supraphysiological thyroid hormone treatment is needed."*

Chen et al. (2004) showed no lower BMD in women with differentiated thyroid cancer treated with

T4 and suppressed TSH levels, but they found low BMD in post-menopausal women with TSH suppression. They did recommend BMD monitoring in the post-menopausal group.

Despite the conflict in studies, the bottom line is that a suppressed TSH but normal T3 and T4 probably is not a cause of reduced BMD. However, monitoring BMD with regular Bone Densitometry and perhaps regular Cross Lap measurements would be good medical practice, especially in the post-menopausal age group.

Another point of view is that if the TSH is suppressed by giving larger doses of T4 to improve patient symptoms, the patient feels better. This leads to increased activity and exercise which could help with weight reduction. Being more active can also help maintain BMD.

Conversely, if lower doses are given, the patient tends to be cold, tired, and sluggish. They gain weight and are less active, and this may affect the bones negatively.

The other point is that post-menopausal women with suppressed TSH tend to do worse, possibly due in part to the osteoporosis associated with menopause.

Overt hyperthyroidism and overt hypothyroidism affect the heart. Excess T3 can cause atrial fibrillation, palpitations, and breathlessness. The excess T3 and not the suppressed TSH cause this.

T3 deficiency in hypothyroidism can cause bradycardia, pericardial effusion, heart failure and coronary atheroma. Less known is that hypothyroidism can produce ventricular dysrhythmias. The thyroid hormone causes all these effects and not the suppressed, or elevated, TSH (Toft & Boon, 2000, Klein & Danzi, 2007).

Shapio et al. (1997) demonstrated that TSH suppression does not have a major effect on the heart. *"Therefore, in the absence of symptoms of thyrotoxicosis, patients treated with TSH-suppressive doses of L-T4 may be followed clinically without specific cardiac laboratory studies."* Here again, the question that needs to be asked; Is it the elevated T3 or the suppressed TSH that is causing the problem? A part of regular monitoring of the patient includes measuring heart rate and blood pressure.

I remember one patient who asked for the dose to be reduced, not because she was feeling over-replaced and unwell but "to keep the endocrinologist happy".

I have heard stories of patients who self-increase their dose to a point where they feel well. They then see their local doctor, who does a blood test and panics when the results come back. The doctor urgently contacts the patient and tells them to reduce the dose because the TSH is suppressed and that they are "taking too much replacement and that could be dangerous". The patient is confused because they feel good/normal at the dose they are taking. Some do reduce the dose and while their blood test comes back to "normal", they report feeling awful with the return of hypothyroid symptoms.

Is the aim then to treat the person optimally so that they feel well? Or do we try to normalise the blood test no matter how they feel?

In this book I aim to show that people can have a "normal blood test" and still have the hypothyroid syndrome. I also aim to show that some people do not adequately respond to T4 alone. If you think about this, these two scenarios are related.

POINTS TO PONDER:

1/ Not every patient responds to levothyroxine (T4) alone.

2/ Patients can have hypothyroid syndrome with normal blood test results.

3/ Some patients may need a TSH suppressive dose of thyroid replacement just to feel well.

4/ TSH suppression does not cause osteoporosis or heart disease as long as levels of T4 and T3 are normal.

5/ Every patient is an individual and may present differently.

Chapter 2
The hypothyroid syndrome

There is a very good reason why I call this the hypothyroid syndrome as you shall see.

A syndrome is defined as *"a combination of symptoms resulting from a single cause or so commonly occurring together as to constitute a distinct clinical picture."*

(https://medical-dictionary.thefreedictionary.com/syndrome)

I call it a "syndrome" because the way hypothyroidism presents aligns with the technical definition of a syndrome. There is a distinctive set of symptoms (see table 1), which, from a clinical point of view, can be related to underactive thyroid function. Orthodox medicine seems to have narrowed down the confirmation of the diagnosis of hypothyroidism to a specific blood test, notably the level of thyroid stimulating hormone (TSH), which, as we will see, may not necessarily be a reliable measurement. Conventional medicine stipulates that if the TSH is normal, then it *cannot* be a thyroid problem, even if all the symptoms are there.

This is where I disagree. Hypothyroidism can occur with normal blood test results.

TSH may not be a reliable measure of thyroid function.

This book is all about why I disagree and explain my point of view.

Table 1

Symptoms of hypothyroidism

- Fatigue or Excessive Tiredness
- Weight Gain
- Obesity
- Cold Extremities
- Swollen Neck or Goitre
- Loss of Stamina
- Afternoon Energy Crash

The Hypothyroid Syndrome

- Low Morning Temperature

- Difficulty Breathing

- Dry and/or Gritty Eyes

- Slow Recovery

- Inability to Exercise

- Trembling, Jittery, or Shivering Feeling

- Hoarse Voice

- Cold Sweats

- Lack of Coordination

- Heavy Eyelids

- Insomnia

- Poor Sleep Quality

- Waking Up Feeling Tired

- Difficulty Getting Out of Bed in the Morning

- Frequent Nightmares

- Sleep Apnoea

- Excessive Snoring

- Night Sweats

- Inability to Concentrate

- Slowed Reflexes and Reaction Time

- Sensitivity to Light and/or Sun

- Sensitivity to Cold

- Sensitivity to Strong Odours

- Sensitivity to Loud Noises

- Blurred Vision

- Puffiness or Swelling of Eyes, Face, Hands, Feet, and/or Ankles

- Hair Loss

- Brittle Hair

- Loss of Eyelashes

- Loss of Eyebrow Hair (outer portion)

- Brittle, Flaky, or Peeling Nails

- Dry, Flaky, or Course Skin

The Hypothyroid Syndrome

- Pale and/or Yellowish Skin Pigment

- Dark Circles Under Eyes

- Orange Calluses

- Bruise Easily

- Acne

- Rashes and Various Skin Conditions

- Loss of Appetite

- Constipation

- Food Allergies and Sensitivities

- Difficulty Swallowing

- Swollen Tongue or Ridges on Tongue

- Dry Mouth

- Alcohol Intolerance

- Haemorrhoids

- Irritable Bowel Syndrome (IBS)

- Abdominal Distention

- Excessive Gas

- Bad Breath

- Diabetes

- Liver/Gallbladder Issues

- Salt Cravings

- Sweet Cravings

- Hypoglycaemia

- High Cholesterol

- High Blood Pressure

- Low Blood Pressure

- Slow/Weak Pulse (under 60 bpm)

- Heart Palpitations

- Heart Disease

- Bleeding/Clotting Issues

- Recurring Urinary Tract Infections (UTIs)

- Recurring Upper Respiratory Infections

- Fungal and Candida Infections

- Rheumatoid Arthritis

- Lupus

- Asthma

- Multiple Sclerosis

- Autoimmune Disease

- Cancer

- Panic attacks

- Poor Memory

- Confusion

- Restlessness

- Mental Sluggishness

- ADD/ADHD

- Slowed Speech

- Difficulty Learning New Things

- Poor Concentration

- Phobias

- Loss of Motivation

- Light Headedness

- Vertigo or Dizziness

- Postpartum Depression

- Epilepsy or Seizures

- Depression

- Nervousness and Anxiety

- Easily Upset

- Antisocial Behaviour

- Mood Swings

- Lack of Confidence

- Bipolar Tendencies

- Migraines

- Pressure Headaches

- Muscle Cramps

- Muscle Spasms

- Back Pain

- Wrist Pain

- Foot Pain

- Arthritis

- Joint Pain or Stiffness

- Carpal Tunnel Syndrome

- Tendinitis

- PMT

- Irregular, Longer, Lighter, or Heavier Menstrual Cycles

- Severe Menstrual Cramps

- Infertility

- History of Miscarriage

- Fibroids

- Loss of Libido (Female and male)

- Erectile Dysfunction

(https://thyroidproofdiet.com › low-thyroid-symptoms)

Of course, not everyone has all these symptoms. Conversely, if you have one of the conditions listed, you may not necessarily have hypothyroidism. The first seven or eight symptoms are the most common. We must look at all the symptoms wholistically. That is, it is important to look at the big picture first, otherwise you may miss the diagnosis.

Some people present to their doctor with the signs and symptoms of hypothyroidism but are not diagnosed as such because their TSH is normal. As orthodox medicine does not have a solution, these people are dismissed, and they continue to suffer. One symptom of hypothyroidism is depression, so it is not unusual for a diagnosis of depression to be made, and an antidepressant medication prescribed. You would also become depressed if you have been feeling unwell for so long and a solution cannot be found.

Another reason I consider this disorder a "syndrome" is because it would cover all the types of hypothyroidism. In any orthodox textbook on thyroid disease, two fundamental types of hypothyroidism are described:

1/ Primary hypothyroidism and

2/ Secondary hypothyroidism.

Primary hypothyroidism is where the problem is with the thyroid gland itself, where the gland is damaged or compromised and cannot produce adequate amounts of thyroid hormone. Examples of this are the autoimmune disease, Hashimoto's thyroiditis, a nutritional deficiency of iodine, or an extreme example, thyroidectomy, where the thyroid gland is surgically removed. A thyroid function test (TFT) generally shows a high TSH and a low thyroxine (T4) level.

Secondary hypothyroidism is where the problem is with the pituitary gland. The pituitary gland produces the thyroid regulating hormone TSH, and this regulates the function of the thyroid gland. For example, a tumour, a micro adenoma can develop in the pituitary and can slowly grow and destroy that part of the pituitary that produces TSH. When enough cells are destroyed then little, or no TSH is produced. Without TSH, there is no stimulation of the thyroid. A TFT generally shows a low TSH and a low T4.

I will not dwell on these types of hypothyroidism as they are well described in most textbooks. However, how I treat all these forms of hypothyroidism is much the same, so to some extent, it doesn't really matter what the diagnosis is. However, I should point out here that if there is a tumour or an iodine deficiency or autoimmunity or any other condition, they, of course, must be addressed in addition to the usual treatment.

What I would like to focus on in this book is one condition that generally is not really recognised by the orthodox medicine, and that is the condition I will call Tertiary Hypothyroidism.

POINTS TO PONDER:

1/ TSH alone may not necessarily be a suitable measurement.

2/ Treat the patient, not the blood test.

3/ Concentrate on the symptoms.

4/ Hypothyroidism can present in many ways. It is more common than you think.

Chapter 3
Tertiary hypothyroidism

This condition has all the signs and symptoms of hypothyroidism, but the problem is **not** with the thyroid gland or the pituitary gland. The problem is with the *peripheral hormone metabolism*. Technically, this can be considered a thyroid problem, as part of the thyroid system is the action of the hormone at the periphery. There is no point to the complex biochemistry that makes a hormone if it cannot be used properly.

In this situation, a normal pituitary gland produces a normal amount of TSH to which the normal thyroid gland responds normally. The thyroid gland produces mainly T4 but also some T3, hence the investigations such as thyroid function tests (TFT), TSH and T4 can be relatively normal. However, T3 measurement can be low. Though it should be noted that T3 levels are not always measured. The problem lies at the periphery where the hormone cannot be processed or used properly at the cellular level. This produces all the signs and symptoms of hypothyroidism, yet the TSH and T4 results can be normal.

This answers the clinical conundrum where the person presents with all or many of the signs of hypothyroidism, yet has normal blood tests. Orthodox doctors dismiss these people. As earlier stated, a "syndrome" is a collection of symptoms; these symptoms are typical of hypothyroidism, *but* blood tests are largely normal. Such a situation certainly does cause problems with doctors and patients because the doctors do not, or cannot, or do not want to diagnose hypothyroidism and the patient continues to suffer.

Thyroid disease can present with a normal TSH.

Those who are dismissed by their doctors inevitably end up searching elsewhere for answers. They consult naturopaths, chiropractors and herbalists or they go to an integrative doctor to find a solution.

There is treatment; the use of nutrients, herbs, and, in the correct situation, thyroid hormone replacement, can bring great relief to those who have been told there is nothing wrong with them. And, while it may sound counter-intuitive, these people can be, and should be treated with appropriate thyroid replacement.

The Hypothyroid Syndrome

Why doesn't or why cannot the doctor diagnose this? The main reason is that this is not part of the orthodox paradigm. Most doctors rely on investigations and tests rather than a thorough clinical assessment that questions and looks further when results are not consistent with the presenting symptoms. For there to be thyroid disease, they believe there needs to be abnormal thyroid test results. Normal thyroid tests, they conclude, equal a non-thyroid condition.

Here I must point out that certain blood tests can be done that may help in diagnosing tertiary hypothyroidism. Unfortunately, these tests are generally not done, and it is possible that many orthodox doctors do not know about these tests! This will be discussed later.

There is a condition that is very similar to tertiary hypothyroidism that mainstream medicine does acknowledge. This is called the "sick euthyroid syndrome (SES)" or otherwise known as "non thyroidal illness". It is called "non-thyroidal illness" as it is not caused by an abnormality of the hypothalamus – pituitary – thyroid (HPT) axis itself, however there is an abnormality in the way the thyroid hormone is utilised. This is the same for tertiary hypothyroidism. I would argue that SES is probably a form of tertiary hypothyroidism.

Yu and Koenig (2000) wrote *"nonthyroidal illness, also known as the sick euthyroid syndrome, is characterized by a low plasma T3 and an "inappropriately normal" plasma thyrotropin (TSH) in the absence of intrinsic disease of the hypothalamic-pituitary-thyroid axis. "*

The researchers discuss the action of cytokines on the activity of the deiodinase type 2 enzyme (DIO2) and in the reduction in the formation of T3.

I was amused by their description of the "inappropriately normal" TSH levels, i.e., a thyroid-like condition with "normal TSH".

The symptoms of SES are the same as hypothyroidism. Some abnormal findings in the TFT characterise the condition, where there is an absence of HPT axis dysfunction. The most common finding is a low T3 because of reduced T4 to T3 conversion.

SES was initially thought to happen only in critically ill patients in an intensive care unit (ICU) scenario and was therefore uncommon, but it is possible that it can happen in people who are sick, stressed and not necessarily in hospital. It is seen in those suffering from various acute and chronic conditions including chronic underlying systemic illnesses such as renal disease, heart disease, lung disease, and gut disease, in metabolic disorders including diabetes, inflammatory conditions, fasting/starvation, and in trauma, including surgery, burns and sepsis, heart attacks, stress and cancer.

If you consider how many people in this world are stressed, suffer inflammation, are diabetic and have chronic diseases, it is not unreasonable to believe that there is so much of this condition about. I, personally, do not believe that we recognise this form of hypothyroidism enough; there are many people with normal blood tests results of TSH and T4 (but remember that T3 is rarely measured) who have the hypothyroid syndrome.

Lee and Farwell (2016) consider SES to be a condition that is an adaptive response to illness. They note that there are *"Multiple mechanisms ... including alterations in the iodothyronine deiodinases, thyroid-stimulating hormone secretion, thyroid hormone binding to plasma protein, transport of thyroid hormone in peripheral tissues, and thyroid hormone receptor activity."*

This concurs with the research on navy divers (McCormack, Reed, Thomas, & Malik, 1996) and mountaineering expeditions (Hackney, Feith, Pozos, & Seale, 1995) which will be discussed further on.

Dr Peter Baratosy MBBS FACNEM

Chapter 4
Hypothyroid diagnosis

"How was thyroid disease diagnosed in the past before blood tests were invented?"

The symptoms of the syndrome of hypothyroidism were first recognised in mid-1800s as relating to the thyroid gland. This connection between the thyroid and the hypothyroid syndrome was discovered after thyroidectomy was performed for goitre or Graves' disease or hyperthyroidism (over-active thyroid). Obviously, not having a thyroid gland produced these symptoms.

As there were no tests to diagnose, how was it diagnosed? With symptoms, of course. There is a consistent combination of symptoms that point to thyroid deficiency.

The Clinical Society of London published a 200-page report in 1888 describing the signs and clinical manifestations of hypothyroidism. Many of these signs and symptoms would still be valid today. (Refer to Table 1.)

My favourite saying to patients:

> If it looks like a duck and walks like a duck and quacks like a duck – it's a duck!

Basing the diagnosis on symptoms would have included those who may have primary, secondary or tertiary hypothyroidism. In many cases the treatment would be the same, or at least very similar.

Why are modern doctors unable to diagnose hypothyroidism without blood tests? What happened to the art of clinical diagnosis? Is it that doing blood tests is much easier? Or is it because of concern about medico-legal aspects of care?

Current orthodox medicine doctrine says that an abnormal blood test result, especially an abnormal TSH, is the only way to diagnose hypothyroidism. There is some research that points to the fact that the TSH may not necessarily be an accurate method of diagnosing hypothyroidism. There are always exceptions. This book is largely about these "exceptions".

According to Ling et al. (2018) the TSH test may be a *convenient* screen for thyroid function, but factors, such as stress, can influence it. The researchers concluded that where there is a *discordance* between their clinical presentation and their TSH level, further tests *need* to be done. Do not just rely on the TSH.

In another paper, the researchers, Sheikh et al. (2018) make the point that *"TSH should not be used as a single marker of thyroid function."*

Koulouri, Moran, Halsall, Chatterjee, and Gurnell (2013) argue that, and I have also mentioned this, most patients with hypothyroidism are straightforward. Their TSH blood test is congruent with their clinical presentation and treatment is also straightforward. They respond well to the conventional treatment, i.e., levothyroxine.

Many times, I see a patient for some other non-thyroidal issue and on usual history taking I discover they are hypothyroid and are on levothyroxine. Of course, I ask the usual question *"How do you feel?"* If the reply is *"I feel really good!"* then I do not bother altering anything, they stay on the levothyroxine. There is no need to change anything unless they want to.

However, if they answer, *"Actually I still feel unwell, cold, tired, and I'm gaining weight...."* I then can start the conversation and do more regarding the thyroid.

When the blood tests are incongruent with the clinical picture, or where the individual results are incongruent with each other - this will need further investigations.

The TSH may be a convenient *screening test* to diagnose hypothyroidism but is not necessarily a good test to *monitor* levothyroxine replacement.

St J O'Reilly (2010) wrote *"The current controversy and patient disquiet began in the early 1970s, when on **theoretical grounds and without proper assessment, the serum thyrotropin (TSH) concentration was adopted as the means of assessing the adequacy of thyroxine replacement. The published literature shows that the serum TSH concentration is a poor indicator of clinical status in patients on thyroxine.** The adequacy of thyroxine replacement should be assessed clinically with the serum T3 being measured, when required, to detect over-replacement."* (Text highlighted by author)

This is reflected by Alevizaki, Mantzou, Cimponeriu, Alevizaki, and Koutras (2005) who concluded that *"TSH may not be a good marker for adequate thyroid hormone replacement therapy"*

Some people do need a replacement dose that suppresses their TSH to get an adequate clinical improvement. It is not enough to monitor TSH only, T4 and especially T3 levels must be tested as well.

Levothyroxine doses may be increased until there is clinical symptomatic remission, even if there is TSH suppression, on the condition that the level of T3 remains in the "normal range".

Toft (2017) concluded that there are three scenarios in treating hypothyroidism:

1/ Make no change to current practice and as a result have many unhappy patients keep coming back and complaining that they are not better.

2/ give adequate doses of T4, to a level of clinical euthyroidism even if there is TSH suppression. Toft writes that this TSH suppression has *not* shown any evidence of osteoporosis or atrial fibrillation, with the proviso that the T3 remains in the "normal range," and,

3/ prescribe a combination of T3 and T4 and there is a likelihood that the biochemistry will go into the "normal range" *and* there will be clinical remission.

In this 2017 paper, Toft suggests the use of T3, in addition to T4, is more likely to reduce the "TSH suppression".

Midgley, Toft, Larich, Dietrich, and Hoermann wrote in 2019 *"It appears that we are witnessing a consequential historic shift in the treatment of thyroid disease, driven by over-reliance on a single laboratory parameter TSH. The focus on biochemistry rather than patient symptom relief should be re-assessed. A joint consideration together with a more personalized approach may be required to address the recent surge in patient complaint rates."*

A person goes to the doctor complaining of a myriad of symptoms, which from a clinical perspective, certainly fits the diagnosis of hypothyroidism. The doctor is astute enough to consider thyroid disease and does thyroid tests and yet, lo and behold, the test comes back as NORMAL. So, the doctor tells the patient that "there is nothing wrong with your thyroid"

Doctor "There is nothing wrong with your thyroid, your tests are normal"

Patient "Then why do I still feel like crap?!"

In my experience this scenario occurs too frequently. Unfortunately, orthodox medicine does not seem to have an answer to this.

In one way, the doctor is right. There may be nothing wrong with the thyroid gland itself. The thyroid is working normally, *but* the question we must ask is, "Why can't the person use the hormone normally?"

That is the issue here.

When considering what might be wrong, we note that the peripheral use of the thyroid hormone (TH) is the key.

The concept of tertiary hypothyroidism can explain these exceptions.

Essentially, there is enough TH floating in the blood (hence normal blood tests) *but* the body has difficulty using the hormone at the cellular level. The thyroid gland producing the hormone is only half of the story. The other half of the story is for the hormone to get to and attach to its receptor to achieve its function.

An analogous situation occurs with type 2 diabetes. Here the issue is *not* an insulin deficiency. Testing insulin levels in type 2 diabetes can show elevated levels of insulin. So then why is the person diabetic if there is adequate insulin flowing in their veins? The situation here is "insulin resistance".

Is there a thyroid hormone resistance? To some extent there is.

There is a reason that the normal level of TH does not work properly. In other hormone situations e.g., insulin and oestrogen, the hormone receptor is on the cell surface, so any hormone in the blood can attach to the cell surface receptor to achieve its function. Just to clarify, there are two types of oestrogen receptors. One is nuclear and the other is on the cell membrane. This accounts for the dual phase action of oestrogen, an immediate action with the receptor on the cell membrane and a slower phase with the nuclear receptor.

Thyroid is different.

Firstly, there are no T4 receptors. The TH receptor is a T3 receptor and only T3 can activate this receptor. T3 receptors are only found inside the cells and only inside the organelles, specifically the mitochondria and the nucleus. Therefore, 1/ T4 needs to get into the cell, 2/ The T4 needs to be converted to T3 and 3/ the T3 needs to enter the mitochondria and/or the nucleus before it can do its job. As you can see, there are barriers for the TH to achieve its actions.

The situation with tertiary hypothyroidism is that the body cannot use the TH properly. This is a suitable time to introduce the concept of *"cellular or tissue hypothyroidism"*. In a paper aptly titled "Why are our hypothyroid patients unhappy? Is tissue hypothyroidism the answer?" published in 2011, Kalra and Khandelwal introduce the concept of *"cellular"* or *"tissue hypothyroidism"*. They confirm that a significant number of patients continue to complain of symptoms despite being *"adequately replaced"* according to blood tests. They pose the question, *"Should we treat patients according to their TSH level, which represents the health of their hypothalamic-pituitary axis, or according to their symptoms, which represent the health of the whole body?"*

We can measure the levels of TH in the blood, but we cannot measure the levels of TH intracellularly. Intracellular T3/T4 level cannot be measured directly but possibly can be judged by symptoms the person is exhibiting. That publication also introduces the idea of using T3 for treatment. Here I must point out that the use of T3 is only needed for those who have minimal response to T4 alone.

> T3 is only needed for those who have minimal response to T4 alone.

Why can people have all the symptoms of hypothyroidism yet have a normal blood test?

The "normal" blood test indicates that the pituitary–thyroid axis works normally. In tertiary hypothyroidism, the pituitary– thyroid axis *does* work normally. As mentioned earlier, the problem is at the end action of the hormone at the periphery.

T3 is rarely measured, unless specifically asked for, and even then, may not always be done. This is because Medicare, which pays for these tests, seem to have the idea that T3 measurement is not important. Perhaps in simple thyroid issues, it is not that necessary but in cases such as those I am describing, I believe it is extremely important.

Consider the scenario below:

I have seen this situation many times. The TFT comes back as;

TSH - Normal

T4 - Normal

The conclusion then, is that all is normal... however, if we measure the T3 and the result is low, or low normal, what would this indicate?

My interpretation is that T4 is not being converted adequately to T3. This person is complaining of hypothyroid symptoms but the TSH and T4 are normal. Since we have already said that T3 is the active hormone, if T4 is not converting to T3 adequately, then this low T3 could be the reason for hypothyroid symptoms. This whole scenario could be missed if the T3 is not measured.

POINTS TO PONDER:

1/ The use of TSH to monitor levothyroxine replacement was introduced in the early 1970s without any proper assessment.

2/ TSH on its own may not be an effective way of diagnosing thyroid disease.

3/ The interpretation of the TSH must take the symptoms into account.

4/ TSH is not a good measurement of levothyroxine replacement.

5/ TSH suppression may be needed to get good clinical results.

Chapter 5
The journey of Timmy the T4

In order to make the concepts mentioned above very easy to understand, this section is written in the format of a story for children.

The journey of Timmy the T4

Timmy the T4 was born in the thyroid gland. The time came for him to leave home and he spent his time floating in the blood stream waiting for his chance to grow up. You see, Timmy hadn't grown up; he was still pre-pubertal and only when he grows up can he actually do what he was predestined for. There are many steps in the process of Timmy growing up.

He first had to cross the great wall, the cell membrane, to start his transformation from Timmy the T4 to Timothy the T3. When he came to the great wall he could not get through. He knew he had to go through the gate, but he could not go through on his own. He knew that he needed the help of Tracy the Transporter.

Finally, he found Tracy and only with her help could he go through the gate, through the cell wall. Once inside the cell, he was still Timmy, still not able to be the active hormone he was destined to be. He knew the next step was to find Donny the Deiodinase enzyme. Donny was the key for Timmy to grow up and become Timothy the T3, the active hormone he was intended to become. Only Timothy could do the job that was his primary role of stimulating the cell to increase the metabolism. Timmy floated about the cell looking for Donny. Finally, Timmy met up with Donny, who along with his partner, Sally Selenium, helped him grow up to become Timothy the T3. Now Timothy could do the job he was born to do. He could meet up with Rachel the Receptor, join with her, and this would set off a chain of events that would lead to the cell being activated. But there were still obstructions. There were two places where Rachel could be–in the mitochondria or in the nucleus of the cell. A wall, not unlike the great wall, guarded both these areas, but here Timothy didn't need the help of Tracy to get through. He was small enough to squeeze through by himself. Finally, Timothy squeezed through the gaps in these secondary walls and found Rachel, joined together with her, and at last fulfilled his predetermined role. The role he was destined to do!

I purposefully wrote this as a children's story so that there is no excuse for not understanding the story of the journey of Timmy the T4.

The Hypothyroid Syndrome

This above story is the journey without any complications. This is the best scenario. However, there are many stages where Timmy's journey could be obstructed.

1/ What if Tracy the Transporter was not working properly? What if Tracy had some form of disability?

2/ What if the great wall was abnormal and impeded Tracy's passage?

3/ What if Donny the Deiodinase was not working properly. What if Donny was disabled?

4/ What if Donny's partner, Sally Selenium was missing, Donny could not work alone.

5/ What if Rachel the Receptor was blocked?

6/ What if the wall that separated Timothy from Rachel was thicker or denser than usual and Timothy had difficulty squeezing through the wall?

All these scenarios could have a delaying effect on Timmy growing up to become Timothy. You could call this a form of "thyroid resistance".

PART 2

Chapter 6
The scientific basis behind the journey of Timmy the T4

Timmy the T4 had many potential obstructions in his journey to become Timothy the T3. We will now explore these possible obstacles.

1/ The role of the thyroid transporter

Initially, the thinking was that the thyroid hormone (TH) crossed the cell membrane by passive diffusion. This idea has been shown to be incorrect. (Visser, 2013) Transporter proteins are needed to carry the TH into the cell. Without this transporter, TH cannot get into the cell and fulfill its role. Many TH transporters have been identified; some are specific such as monocarboxylate 8 (MCT 8), and some are nonspecific. A rare syndrome called the Allan Herndon Dudley syndrome clearly illustrates the importance of thyroid transporters.

Schweizer and Köhrle (2013) discuss this syndrome, which is a very rare X chromosome linked moderate to severe intellectual disability disorder, and result from a mutation in the thyroid transporter, monocarboxylate transporter 8 (MCT8) gene. Normal TH function is required for normal brain development and as the TH cannot be transported into the cell, especially the brain, brain development is compromised while in utero. This concept is supported by Bernal, Guadaño-Ferraz, and Morte (2015).

Reduced TH transport into the cells is also associated with a wide range of conditions including insulin resistance, diabetes, depression, bipolar disorder, hyperlipidaemia, chronic fatigue syndrome, fibromyalgia, neurodegenerative disease, migraine, stress, anxiety, chronic dieting, and ageing (Holtorf, 2014). What we do not know is if this is a cause or a result.

Since the pituitary has different transporters, pituitary function remains unchanged. Thus, the normal feedback loop is maintained while the rest of the body suffers from cellular hypothyroidism. Serum TH levels do not necessarily correlate with cellular levels. The thyroid transporters are highly energy dependant and therefore may be affected where energy production is compromised, such as with toxins, mitochondrial dysfunction, and dieting (Holtorf, 2014).

What is not known is the reason there is this reduced function of the transporters. Is it due to interference with energy production, an effect on the transporter itself, inflammation, or an effect on the cell membrane or some combination of these?

2/ The role of the cell membrane

A double layer of phospholipids, where the water-soluble heads (hydrophilic) are facing outwards and the lipid soluble (hydrophobic) tails are facing inwards, makes the cell membrane, also known as the plasma membrane. This double layer of phospholipids makes up the cell walls as well as the walls of the various organelles in the cell. Within this double layer there are fats which give the cell wall its specific characteristics and proteins which act as receptors or carrier proteins. Cholesterol and saturated fats make the cell wall more solid, while poly unsaturated fatty acids (PUFA) such as eicosapentaenoic acid (EPA), docosahexaenoic acid (DHA) and arachidonic acid (AA) make the cell wall more "fluid". This composition of the cell membrane influences cell wall fluidity, receptor function, transporter function, cell signalling mechanisms, membrane-bound enzymes and regulation of eicosanoid synthesis and gene expression (Spector & Yorek, 1985).

In other words, the cell wall must be strong

enough to prevent cell breakdown and to prevent just any molecule gaining entry to the cell but fluid enough to regulate diffusion of important molecules into the cell, to prevent harmful molecules getting in, to allow carrier proteins to move through the walls and for receptors to function properly (Clamp, Ladha, Clark, Grimble, & Lund, 1997). Basically, the transporters do not work as well as intended if the cell membrane is abnormal.

Hulbert, Turner, Storlien, and Else (2005) showed that the cell membrane has a relatively stable content of saturated and monounsaturated fats over a wide variation of dietary intake. However, they also showed that the greatest response to cell membrane changes was to omega 3 and omega 6 levels in the diet.

The modern western diet is full of the wrong fats. We eat *too* many plant-based omega 6 fatty acids (corn, sunflower, safflower, canola oils) and too many trans fatty acids (TFA), margarines and hydrogenated fats. At the same time, we eat inadequate omega 3 fatty acids, notably fish, which is high in DHA. Another important dietary factor needed for proper cell membrane function is cholesterol… and we know how badly cholesterol is maligned.

Our ancestors ate a diet with an omega 3 to omega 6 ratio of 1:1 to 1:2. The animals that they hunted had a higher omega 3 content and a lower omega 6 content because they were "free range": these animals ate what they were designed to eat.

In current western diets, the ratio is abnormally high in favour of the omega 6. The omega 3 to omega 6 ratio can be as high as 1:20 to1:40. We eat *too* much omega 6 and not enough omega 3. Today's meat and eggs have a higher omega 6 level and lower omega 3 level because these animals are fed on high omega 6 grains, which is NOT their natural food. "Free range", "grass fed" meat has a more normal omega 3 to omega 6 ratio. This does not mean that omega 6 is bad in itself, it is only "bad" when out of proportion to omega 3.

For example, deficiency of DHA can influence thyroid, as well as insulin and oestrogen receptor function. The bottom line is that if the membrane is abnormal, it will not work as intended. This abnormal cell membrane will have difficulty in allowing TH into the cell due to the effect on the transporters.

As we age the cell walls become stiff and viscous, as fats oxidise, and damaged lipids accumulate in the cell walls. Consequently, our cell membranes do not function as well as they should. Kurtas (2016) states that antioxidants can be helpful by protecting the cell walls and maintaining function.

Pritchard (1979) showed that cells membranes can be disrupted by various toxins, such as heavy metals, pesticides, and xenobiotics. Ginter and Simko (2016) showed that trans fatty acids (TFA) have a negative effect on the cell membrane.

Dietary fat consumption does have a bearing on cell membrane structure (Ibarguren, López, & Escribá, 2014). So, part of treating tertiary hypothyroidism is to improve the diet, which means improving the omega 3 to omega 6 ratio, to remove the trans fatty acids, and remove toxins, pesticides and heavy metals. This can be achieved by changing to an organic and free-range diet. Kis, Varga, and Lugasi (2006) and Hallmann (2012) have shown that organic foods have fewer chemicals and pesticides and other residuals than non-organic foods. Also, it may be a good idea to use a water filter, specifically a reverse osmosis unit, to remove any toxins, fluoride, and heavy metals from the water.

3/ Deiodinase issues

The enzyme that converts T4 to T3 is deiodinase type 2 (DIO2). There are three types of deiodinases and to keep the discussion simple, I will not be going into too many details. DIO 2 removes an iodine from T4 to produce T3. Another deiodinase, type 3 (DIO3) removes an iodine from a different position and forms reverse T3 (rT3), an inactive isomer of T3. I will discuss rT3 later. Another important facet of the deiodinases is that they are a *selenium dependant* enzyme. I will discuss selenium in the next section.

Without an optimally functioning DIO2, the T4 cannot be converted to the active thyroid hormone, T3.

There are factors that can affect the function of the deiodinases.

Singh et al. (2014) showed that environmental factors, such as fluoride, have a negative effect on the function of the deiodinases. Fluoride is a toxic element that is purposefully put into the drinking water (Shashi & Singla, 2013).

Peckham, Lowery, and Spencer (2015) performed a large observational study of GP practice data looking at hypothyroidism incidence and fluoride levels in the drinking water and showed that there was a higher incidence of hypothyroidism in areas that were fluoridated than in areas that were less fluoridated or not at all. This study, however, did not specifically look at the mechanism of how the fluoride produced the hypothyroidism.

However, in a review of the action of fluoride on the thyroid, Gill (2014) showed that fluoride can interfere with thyroid function in many ways:

1/ fluoride interferes with iodine uptake,

2/ fluoride is a G-protein activator/inhibitor,

3/ fluoride is a TSH analogue,

4/ fluoride inhibits thyroid hormone transport,

5/ fluoride interferes with deiodinases.

Inflammation affects the workings of the deiodinases. This is a tissue level problem. Mancini et al. (2016) and Elnagar, Abdel-Salam Dawood, and Abdelwahab Elshewy (2018) showed that inflammation and oxidative stress alter the conversion of T4 to T3. Inflammation is a big problem and is possibly one of the main underlying factors in nearly all diseases. Dealing with inflammation is an important part of treating thyroid disease, and any other chronic diseases for that matter.

Another reason for deiodinase problems is genetic. There is a group of people who inherit a single nucleotide polymorphism (SNP – called a "snip") of the deiodinase Type 2 (DIO2) enzyme. A SNP is a genetic mutation/variation where one amino acid in the protein chain is different. This causes the protein to have different properties. If the protein is an enzyme, a SNP in a non-critical area would produce virtually no effects. However, if the SNP is in a critical area, the protein chain folds into a different shape which does alter the action of the enzyme.

Remember: protein structure/shape equals function.

Panicker et al. (2009) showed in their research that this DIO2 variation was present in 16% of their study population. This variant enzyme is not as active as the "normal" enzyme, therefore has difficulty with peripheral conversion of T4 to T3. The vast majority of T3 production-80%-is T4 to T3 conversion by the DIO2 enzyme intracellularly. This group of people with the DIO2 SNP are possibly the ones who do better on T3/T4 combination than T4 alone because of the poor peripheral conversion.

McDermott (2012) stated that most hypothyroid people do well on T4 only, however because of poor peripheral conversion, those with the DIO2 SNP are the ones that do better with the combination of T4 and T3.

Unfortunately, at present, the ability of clinicians to test for this SNP is unavailable. Many companies offer genetic testing, but this gene is not one that is included. We can assume that if the person is not responding adequately to T4 only, then the addition of T3 would be an appropriate and logical thing to do.

Dietary fats also can be problematic. The long-chained poly unsaturated fatty acids (PUFA) such as arachidonic acid, linolenic acid, linoleic acid, and oleic acid have an inhibiting effect on T4 to T3 conversion. Other lipids have little or no such action. (Chopra et al., 1985)

4/ The role of selenium

Selenium is a trace mineral that is generally very low in Australian soils (Lyons et al., 2005). If the soil levels are low in selenium, then so are the fruits and vegetables that are grown in that soil. Also, the meat and eggs of the animals that eat the plants are also low in selenium. This important because as stated above, selenium is a co-factor in the deiodinase enzymes. Arthur, Nicol, and Beckett (1993) and Wu, Xia, and Chen (1995) showed that a selenium deficiency does have a negative impact on the deiodinase function.

As Australian soils are largely deficient in selenium, it follows that a large part of the Australian population is selenium deficient, or at least very low. I maintain that in Australia, if selenium is *not* supplemented, then there is probably a deficiency.

A particularly toxic element that has a negative effect on selenium levels is mercury. Mercury is the most toxic non-radioactive element known. However, if all elements are considered, mercury is the second most toxic element, the first being plutonium.

In the polluted western society, mercury is a quite common toxin. This includes, not necessarily in any particular order:

* Seafood, in any form, fish and shellfish, as the oceans are heavily polluted with mercury. Fish in rivers

especially if there are factories nearby are also heavily polluted. Little fish are eaten by bigger fish, and they are eaten by even bigger fish. Pollutants, such as mercury, tend to accumulate in the bigger fish. Avoid big, top of the food chain fish. Eat the smaller fish e.g., sardines.

*Dental amalgams are also a source, though the use of dental amalgam is being slowly phased out.

*A preservative, thiomersal, found in various pharmaceuticals, including vaccines, is another source, although this has been almost completely phased out.

*Fluorescent light tubes and the "energy saving" bulbs contain mercury. Be wary if ever you break one of these! It would be advisable to have a Hazmat team to clean up the mercury.

*Coal fired power stations. Burning coal releases the mercury and the exhausts from these power stations contain mercury. Try not to live downwind from a power station.

* Mercury and lead were components of paints. Mercury was used as an antifungal and as a colouring agent as recently as 1990 when it was banned in the USA. Renovating old building, sanding of old paints could lead to mercury and lead poisoning if proper precautions are not taken. Agosc et al. (1990) showed that just by living in homes painted with old mercury containing latex paints can also be hazardous.

In a study by Ye et al. (2016), on average, the mean mercury blood level in humans is 1–8 µg /L, while in urine is 4–5 µg /L. The levels in the human body should be zero.

Mercury is so toxic that there are really NO safe levels.

Spiller (2018) showed that mercury has a negative effect on selenium levels. Mori et al. (2006) have shown that mercury can have a negative influence on the action of the deiodinases and therefore affect the conversion of T4 to T3 thus producing cellular hypothyroidism.

As well as mercury, other heavy metals, such as lead (Pb) and cadmium (Cd) can also produce a negative effect on thyroid function (Rezaei et al., 2019).

Heavy metals can be tested for, and if present, can be removed with chelation therapy. Compounds such as ethylene diamine tetra acetic acid (EDTA) and di mercapto succinic acid (DMSA) can be used to help eliminate the heavy metals.

I made mention of reverse T3 (rT3) earlier. rT3 is an isomer of T3. It has the same chemical formula but has a different configuration of attached iodines. It is an inactive molecule.

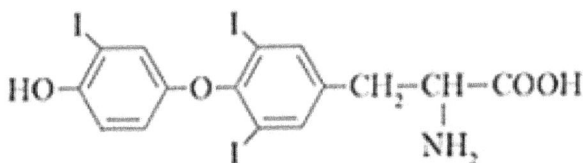

T3

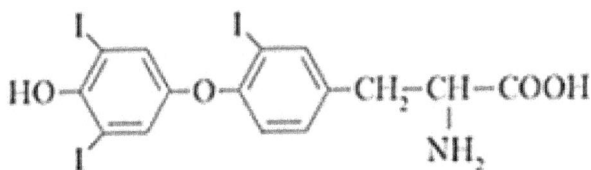

rT3

rT3 is made when T4 is converted to rT3
by the DIO3 enzyme.

In a review of peripheral thyroid hormone metabolism, Kelly (2000) showed that cortisol produced during times of stress enhances the action of DIO3. It goes without saying that we live in a very stressful world. Under stress, there is a higher incidence of T4 being converted to rT3 with a subsequent reduction of T3. When there is a high level of rT3, there is competitive inhibition of the conversion of T4 to T3, meaning that rT3 has an action on DIO2 and prevents T4 being converted to T3.

Okamoto and Leibfritz (1997) did show that rT3 can cause a peripheral blockage to T3; perhaps it is occupying the T3 receptors without stimulating them.

Overall, rT3 can be considered to a T3 antagonist.

What is the function of rT3? Why does the body make some rT3 continually? All complex mechanisms have a positive and negative influences to produce fine control. Have you ever seen a car with only an accelerator? Or just a brake? rT3 acts as a brake on the peripheral thyroid metabolism. T3 is the accelerator.

High levels of rT3 can benefit the body during times of stress or starvation because it slows metabolism and aids survival.

In a study by McCormack, Reed, Thomas, and Malik (1996) on navy personnel exposed to cold stress in Alaska by the US Navy, blood tests showed increased levels of rT3 and reduced levels of T3.

In another study published in 1995, Hackney, Feith, Pozos, and Seale wrote, *"Moreover, the reduction in T3 was inversely correlated with the rT3 increase .... The findings demonstrate that the resting concentrations of thyroid hormones are disrupted by a mountaineering expedition, specifically an environmental stress-related "low T3 condition" seems to develop. These changes would seem to be related to an impaired peripheral conversion of T4 to T3, possibly brought about by elevations in the circulating cortisol levels."*

In summary, stress (and who does not suffer stress in this current world?) enhances the formation of rT3 which then has a negative action on T3, by inhibiting T4 to T3 conversion and possibly by acting as a peripheral T3 receptor blocker to reduce cellular metabolism.

We can measure rT3 in the blood, but this test is generally not done by orthodox doctors. As we cannot measure rT3 intracellularly, serum rT3 possibly can be a good proxy. In my experience, measuring serum rT3 can be useful in understanding and managing patients with complex thyroid problems. See case study pg. 83.

5/ Thyroid receptor blockage

We have already looked at the action of rT3 which can have a blocking effect at the thyroid receptor level. As well as rT3, there are other thyroid receptor blockers.

Research by Wiersinga, Chopra, and Teco (1988) has shown that unsaturated long chained fatty acids (PUFA) have an inhibiting effect on T3 nuclear binding. *"Unsaturated fatty acids were potent inhibitors of the binding of [125I] T3 to isolated rat liver nuclei."* The unsaturated fatty acids included palmitoleic acid, linoleic acid, oleic acid, arachidonic acid, and linolenic acid. Other lipids had little or no inhibitory activity.

This is confirmed by Yammoto Li, Mita, Morisawa, and Inoue (2001), Inoue et al. (1989) and Wiersinga, Chopra, and Teco (1988).

Although not specifically included in this category, long chained unsaturated fatty acids can also interfere with T4 binding to thyroxine binding globulin (TBG), while saturated fatty acids do not. TBG is the protein that transports T3 and T4 in the blood stream. What is bound to TBG is biologically unavailable. Only the "free T4 and T3" can be transported into the cells. This would influence peripheral thyroid function and can cause a general thyroid problem (Tabachnick & Korcek, 1986).

PART 3

Chapter 7
Treatment: preliminary considerations

There are many similarities in treating hypothyroidism, whether it is primary, secondary, or tertiary. The discussion here will be about how to approach hypothyroidism in general and this could apply to all forms of hypothyroidism.

Treating hypothyroidism is not just replacing hormones. Possibly one reason why so many with hypothyroidism do not get the full benefit of treatment is because only hormones are replaced. The thyroid is not an organ functioning on its own; it works in conjunction with many other systems, and therefore any problems must be considered from a wholistic point of view. If we do not address the other systems, then we are only partly treating the condition.

The thyroid is intricately connected to the adrenal system. The thyroid affects the adrenals, and the adrenals affect the thyroid. Earlier we saw that stress/cortisol influences the DIO3, increasing levels of rT3, which can block the conversion of T4 to T3.

Adrenal issues need to be considered and, where necessary, treated.

The thyroid is also closely connected to the gut. There are many gut symptoms not necessarily related to the lack of thyroid hormone *per se*, however the gut needs to be treated as well as the thyroid.

The majority of hypothyroidism occurs in women. The thyroid affects the female hormone system; the female hormone system affects the thyroid.

If hypothyroidism is to be optimally treated, then an all-system approach is necessary.

As I have called hypothyroidism the "Hypothyroid Syndrome" it follows that treatment is based on the signs and symptoms of the condition. Hypothyroidism can present in many ways (Table 1), and doctors need to be vigilant otherwise the condition may be missed.

Relying on blood tests alone could lead to misdiagnosis. An abnormal blood test result more than likely could indicate a thyroid condition; however, a normal test does not necessarily exclude one. Hopefully, you read this book and realised that diagnosing and treating the thyroid is not as simple as it is purported to be, you need to remain open minded. Remember the mind is like an umbrella – it only works when it is open.

The first rule

Treat the person and not the blood test results. This is one of the main guiding principles.

If you remember nothing else but this, you will be way ahead of your peers in treating your patient.

TREAT THE PERSON, NOT THE BLOOD TEST RESULTS.

Get a good history first before doing anything else. Assess the person, ask questions. Do a thorough examination. Use blood tests as a backup but do not rely on them as the sole reason for diagnosis.

The following case study reflects the above principles.

A lady presented with the following thyroid function test results.

	Result	Units	*Ref.Range
Triiodothyronine [Free T3]	8.5*H	pmol/L	3.5 - 6.5
Free Thyroxine [Free T4]	24.6	pmol/L	9.0 - 25.0
Thyroid Stimulating Hormone [TSH]	<0.01*L	mIU/L	0.35 - 5.50

She had seen an endocrinologist who wanted to put her on thyroid suppression medication. The thyroid function test (TFT) does show a suppressed TSH and a high T3 and a high normal T4. A typical result for *hyperthyroidism.* However, on taking her history, she was complaining of being cold, tired, putting on weight and constipated, i.e., all the symptoms of *hypothyroidism.* I wondered if the endocrinologist actually took her clinical history.

How can we explain a blood test that shows hyperthyroidism with symptoms of hypothyroidism? She came to me for a second opinion. After taking a thorough history and performing a comprehensive physical examination, I did one extra test that had not been done, a test I thought would be relevant, a reverse T3 (rT3) test. This came back as extremely high-in fact, the highest I have ever seen. She was under extreme stress, so I started treating her stress advising relaxation, meditation, and gentle exercise. Her diet was terrible, so I gave dietary advice. I started her on adrenal herbs as well as vitamins and minerals, especially selenium. Despite having a high T3, I treated her with slow release T3 (SR T3). Gradually she improved. The hypothyroid symptoms resolved and her TFT normalised.

There are two reasons I treated her with SR T3 even though her T3 was already high. 1/ she was showing signs and symptoms of hypothyroidism and 2/

she has a very high rT3.

The second rule

Treating hypothyroidism is not just replacing thyroid hormone, although it can be a major part.

TREATING HYPOTHYROIDISM IS NOT JUST REPLACING THYROID HORMONE.

I reiterate that it is essential to treat the person from a wholistic point of view. What other symptoms are present? What other complaints are present? These also need to be treated. Many of these symptoms may be related to the hypothyroidism itself, but not necessarily all. Therefore, just replacing the hormone may not specifically address all the complaints.

Firstly, we must ask ourselves, "Is there an adrenal problem?" As stress is a widespread problem in today's world, consider the person's stress levels. We have already discussed that stress/cortisol influences the peripheral conversion of T4 to T3. This is also possibly a good opportunity to measure rT3 level. So, it is important to take a close look at the thyroid-adrenal connection and to provide adrenal support if it is needed.

I do find that adrenal support is nearly always needed, therefore, I routinely prescribe a "Thyroid and Adrenal" nutrition and herb formula for all my thyroid patients.

Chapter 8
The thyroid/adrenal connection

Adrenal gland treatment must be considered in the treatment of thyroid conditions.

There are two adrenal glands, which are pyramid shaped structures, approximately the size of a Brazil nut, one sitting on each of the kidneys (Ad=on and renal=kidney). The main hormones secreted are *adrenalin* from the adrenal medulla, the inner part of the gland and *cortisol*, secreted from the adrenal cortex, the outer portion of the gland. The sympathetic nervous system controls the medulla, while a hormone released from the pituitary, adreno-cortico-trophic hormone (ACTH) controls the cortex.

The term "adrenal fatigue" or "adrenal exhaustion" has been debated about for quite some time. It is a diagnosis made by integrative and complementary doctors, chiropractors and naturopaths. This diagnosis describes a collection of symptoms such as tiredness, poor immunity, sleeping difficulties, feeling tired when waking up, unrefreshed sleep, sugar and salt craving, non-specific digestive problems, needing a coffee hit to get started .... and many more. The symptoms are all non-specific. The cluster of symptoms is reminiscent of a low cortisol scenario, though there are overlapping symptoms of hypothyroidism. Stress does seem to play a major role ... and who does not have stress in this modern world of ours?

Those who first coined the terms adrenal fatigue/exhaustion did so after observing and then postulating that under excessive stress the adrenal glands become "fatigued", "tired out" from overwork. When this happens, they cannot produce adequate cortisol that is necessary to keep the body functioning normally.

Note that this is *not* adrenal failure, that is a condition called Addison's disease. However, the symptoms of "adrenal fatigue" are a mild approximation of the symptoms of Addison's disease.

When confronted with a stressful situation, the adrenal glands produce adrenaline and cortisol in the "Fight and Flight" reaction. This goes back to our cave dweller days; the scenario typically is related that our cave dweller ancestor walking through the forest meets up with a sabre-toothed tiger. The acute stress mechanism kicks in; initially releasing adrenaline, then the cortisol kicks in so that the cave dweller can run faster and fight harder. This is a short-term response and once he gets away, things settle down until the next encounter.

This same mechanism is at work today. However, we do not have sabre-toothed tigers. Instead, we have bosses, tax departments, BAS, GST, parking meters, traffic lights, traffic congestion, pollution, EMF, poor diet, relationship breakdowns and are "over worked and under paid" - all stressful. Also, we humans are particularly good at worrying about things that may never actually happen. The same acute stress reaction experienced by our ancestors kicks in, but we cannot run or fight. For most people it is a matter of just putting up with it, and this probably makes things worse, as it becomes a cause of frustration and even anxiety. We could run and fight, but I do not think it would be a good idea to punch the boss. The stressful events experienced today are more continuous, and our bodies were not designed for such constant stress. As humans have not developed a chronic stress mechanism, the body uses the acute stress mechanism repeatedly.

The various World Endocrinological Societies have never accepted the concept of "adrenal exhaustion". These societies put out statements that "adrenal fatigue" or "adrenal exhaustion" is all a load of rubbish, a figment of the "alternative medicine" mind. The adrenal glands, they assert, *do not* "wear out".

Although they do not offer any explanation for these symptoms, they do say that other diseases must be ruled out.

All good doctors will do this anyway.

The complementary and integrative doctors maintain that since the diagnosis is not being recognised, the diagnosis is not being made and many people with these symptoms do not get any relief from the orthodox approach. So, the people with these symptoms go to alternative practitioners, get diagnosed with "adrenal fatigue", are treated, and greatly improve.

Luckily, the treatment is much the same no matter what you call it.

There is another condition called burnout syndrome, which is quite prominent in the psychological literature. In a paper by Pranjić, Nuhbegović, Brekalo-Lazarević, and Kurtić (2012) the condition is not explained nor assigned any physiology or biochemistry. It is diagnosed on symptoms and questionnaires alone. The symptoms are similar to "adrenal fatigue".

Symptoms

- Adrenal Exhaustion
- Depression/anxiety
- Gut issues
- Lack of energy
- Difficulty getting off to sleep
- Difficulty waking up
- Aches and pains
- Decreased ability to handle stress
- Low body temperature
- Hair loss
- Dizziness

- Burnout Syndrome
- Anxiety/Depression/loss of motivation
- Loss of enjoyment
- Stomach issues
- Decreased energy
- Difficulty getting off to sleep
- Headaches
- Muscle and back pain
- Eating more or less than usual
- Raised heart rate
- Skin flare ups

Above slide taken from a presentation the author gave to the Australian Medical Acupuncture College seminar in 2018.

This syndrome is largely related to stress and work. According to the paper referred to above (Pranjić, Nuhbegović, Brekalo-Lazarević, & Kurtić, 2012), from a symptomatic point of view, there is a great overlap between the symptoms of "adrenal fatigue" and burnout syndrome. Orthodox medicine is more accepting of burnout syndrome as a valid condition rather than "adrenal fatigue".

Can both sides be right? To an extent–yes. Mainly because the issue is *all in the name*. As William Shakespeare wrote in *Romeo and Juliet,* Act 2, Scene 2, *"A Rose by any other name would smell as sweet.'*

It is all in the name.

A review by Cadegiani and Kater (2016) concluded that "adrenal fatigue" does not exist because all the authors of all the studies reviewed, agreed that the adrenal glands do *not tire out and produce less cortisol.* In some, they detected a low cortisol level, in others a high cortisol level, but in the majority, there was not much change.

The adrenal glands are a robust organ and are able to produce cortisol even after long stressful periods. So how can both sides of the argument be somewhat correct?

There is no doubt that stress does affect our health.

Perhaps we should look at it from a more wholistic perspective.

But before we do this, let's get back to basics.

An understanding of how the stress system, the hypothalamus-pituitary-adrenal axis (HPA) works, is helpful. The HPA axis releases hormones in a circadian rhythm to regulate daily energy needs. The following process is circular. Corticotropin releasing hormone (CRH) is released from the suprachiasmatic nucleus in the hypothalamus, which acts on the pituitary gland to release adrenocorticotropic hormone (ACTH), which then acts on the adrenal glands to release cortisol. In normal individuals, the cortisol release is highest in the mornings and gradually declines by night-time. The release of cortisol in this way gives us the energy to wake up and get moving and provides the energy we need for any daytime activities, with the gradual decline by night-time allowing us to fall asleep. This cycle continues day after day.

The amygdala is the part of the brain that detects stress and physical danger whether real or imagined. It sends a signal to the hypothalamus. From here the sympathetic nervous system sends messages via the autonomic nervous system to release adrenaline from the adrenal glands. This is the immediate stress response. Then the HPA axis kicks in and via the mechanism described previously CRH -> ACTH -> cortisol release to provide a more sustained response. Next, via a negative feedback mechanism, cortisol feeds back to reduce CRH and ACTH production. This feedback mechanism is typical of other systems in the body e.g., the thyroid and TSH. This all happens in the normal situation. However, because of the constant stress in today's world, we do *not* live in a "normal" situation.

With the high stress and the constant release of cortisol, it is not that the adrenal "fatigues" or "tires out" …. rather it is the HPA axis that develops the problem. The HPA axis does not like the constant cortisol stimulation so it *"switches off"*.

Chronically elevated cortisol levels can cause damage, so the body tries to reduce the levels. The body tries to protect itself in several ways.

One way is by developing a cortisol receptor resistance.

The same protective mechanism happens elsewhere in the body in various conditions.

Consider type 2 diabetes.

In type 2 diabetes, the pancreas does not wear out. It is not the pancreas that fatigues; the body develops insulin resistance. In type 2 diabetes, the insulin levels can be high, not low. Can this be like what happens in the stress response? It seems so as it is not the adrenal glands that fatigue, rather it is the HPA axis and the cortisol receptors that are the site of the dysfunction.

In summary, most with "adrenal fatigue" do not necessarily have low cortisol levels. They may have low *"free"* cortisol levels but not necessarily low *"total"* cortisol levels.

Note that at least 80% of the cortisol is bound to

corticosteroid binding globulin (CBG) and another 10% is bound to albumin. Only a small portion is unbound and therefore "free" and only the "free" cortisol is biologically active. The low "free" cortisol produces the symptoms of low cortisol.

One alternative way of measuring cortisol is with a saliva test. However, this only measures the *"free"* cortisol NOT the total cortisol. If both the saliva cortisol and the total cortisol are measured, you may find that the total cortisol may not necessarily be low, it may actually be high, but the "free" cortisol may be low.

Even if the cortisol is low, it is not necessarily due to the adrenal glands not making it, i.e., being fatigued, it is due to a down-regulation of the HPA axis.

Essentially, it can be viewed as a protective mechanism.

One mechanism, as mentioned above, is the development of cortisol receptor resistance (Cohen et al., 2012, Merkulov, Merkulova, & Bondar, 2017).

There can also be an increased level of CBG which reduces the "free" cortisol by binding more (Chan, Carrell, Zhou, & Read, 2013, Mattos et al., 2013, Verhoog et al., 2014).

The level of cortisol can also be reduced by converting the more active cortisol to the less active cortisone, by activation of *11 β-hydroxysteroid dehydrogenase type 2* (11β-HSD2).

Prigent, Maxime, and Annane (2003) showed that 11β-HSD2 can be upregulated by Interleukins such as IL-2, IL-4 and IL-13.

Maydych, Claus, Watzl, and Kleinsorge (2018) showed that Interleukins are increased in inflammation and in stress.

11β-HSD2 can also be upregulated by the hormone dehydroepiandrosterone (DHEA), which also increases the conversion of cortisol to cortisone. (Balazs, Schweizer, Frey, Rohner-Jeanrenaud, & Odermatt, 2008) Note that DHEA can be considered as an adrenal hormone.

Morgan et al. (2004) showed that DHEA levels do rise in acute stress. Maninger, Capitanio, Mason, Ruys, and Mendoza (2010) showed that in rhesus monkeys, DHEA increases in chronic stress as well as acute stress. Humans are probably similar.

All this is a protective mechanism. As the body tries to adapt to chronically high cortisol levels, it may actually overshoot and may produce a low "free" cortisol level. And/or if the cortisol resistance the body acts as if the cortisol is low, resulting in the typical symptoms of a "low cortisol" state.

Therefore, when there is HPA axis dysregulation, the symptoms look the same as if the adrenals are fatigued. The actual problem lies with the regulatory controls, not the "fatigue" of the end organ.

The main causes of HPA axis dysregulation are:

1/ Stress – real or perceived. Any kind of stress can cause the dysregulation, and not only negative stress. Even good stress, eustress, can be a problem if it becomes chronic. Modern living, poor diet, pollution, and other factors that may seem normal can, and do, cause stress,

2/ Inflammation, and

3/ Blood sugar – high or low.

As mentioned earlier, when considering thyroid problems, it is necessary to also consider all systems in the body. It is particularly important to evaluate adrenal function, as those with low adrenal function can have a co-existing thyroid problem. The "adrenal exhaustion" can contribute to the extent of thyroid problem. Remember that these systems work hand in hand.

The elevated cortisol that is part of the stress response has a profound effect on thyroid function.

Cortisol can interfere with the thyroid at different levels:

1/ Cortisol can have an effect at the periphery as already discussed. Cortisol enhances DIO3 which converts T4 to reverse T3 (rT3), an inactive molecule. The increase in rT3 can have a blocking effect on T4 to T3 conversion.

2/ Cortisol can influence anterior pituitary hormones other than ACTH. Rubello et al. (1992) showed that acute cortisol increase does not seem to influence TSH secretion, however chronic cortisol exposure has an inhibiting effect on TSH release caused by an impaired response to thyroid releasing hormone (TRH).

Samuels and McDaniel (1997) showed that cortisol can cause a decrease in TSH levels. *"...these data show that near-physiological doses of HC* (hydrocortisone, same as cortisol) *and resulting changes in serum cortisol levels within the normal range can cause significant decreases in serum TSH levels."*

3/ Cortisol can influence biosynthesis and release of TRH from the hypothalamus. (Kakuscka, Qi, & Lechan, 1995)

If cortisol influences TSH secretion, doesn't this put the usefulness of TSH measurement into doubt?

Stress levels in today's society are very high. In the last few years especially with the pandemic, the lockdowns, the mask wearing, the loss of jobs and shut down of small business, the lockdown of entire countries and so much more, stress levels are constantly high for many people.

Above, I have outlined how stress leads to high cortisol levels, which can lead to interference in TSH release.

High cortisol levels cause T4 to be converted to reverse T3 (rT3), which can block T4 to T3 and produce a functional T3 deficiency.

If the T4 to T3 conversion is deficient, the clinical picture is one of hypothyroidism WITH normal TSH levels.

Normal thyroid function is needed for normal adrenal function. Stress causes increased energy expenditure and an increase in blood sugar level (BSL). In the chronic situation, stress can cause a drop in BSL, which is a signal for cortisol production. Hypothyroidism itself can cause a drop in BSL.

Hypothyroidism produces stress in the body. The

body then needs more cortisol. However, as hypothyroidism also causes a reduction in energy in all tissues, including the adrenal glands, this limits the ability to produce cortisol. So, you can see that thyroid and adrenals do work together.

There are times when, unfortunately, things get even more complicated. The patient complains of coldness, tiredness and other typical signs and symptoms of hypothyroidism. They may even have a low temperature. Clinically, this looks like hypothyroidism, however, when treated with levothyroxine, DT or SR T3, *they may even get worse*.

What is going on here?

It is in this phase of "adrenal exhaustion" that giving thyroid replacement can make matters worse. The patient usually says, *"I felt worse on the thyroid replacement, so I stopped it".*

Unfortunately, it is not always easy to diagnose this situation initially. If a patient presents with a history that they had already adversely reacted to thyroid treatment, then it is probably mandatory to test for and treat the "adrenal exhaustion" first.

There are a few clues that could alert you to this situation.

Bear this in mind when

1/ the whole case is not typical, or

2/ when things are "not quite right" or

3/ when the illness has been *long drawn out* or

4/ when there has been *excessive* stress, or

5/ when the history shows a mixed picture – i.e., signs and symptoms of both hyper and hypothyroidism.

While there are some clinical signs of "adrenal exhaustion", they are very subtle.

1/ The blood pressure is excessively low. There may even be a drop in BP on standing from the sitting position (postural hypotension). This can be easily tested by measuring BP in the sitting then in the standing position. This produces the symptom of dizziness on standing, or dizziness on prolonged standing. Normally BP rises on standing.

2/ The pupil reflex is slow, unstable, or even reversed.

3/ Tendon reflexes may be abnormal, especially the Achilles reflex. The actual reflex is normal, but the relaxation phase is prolonged, i.e., slow relaxation.

Testing for "adrenal exhaustion" is not easy. Conventional tests, such as the 24-hour urinary cortisol which involves collecting all urine in a 24-hour period, are not very accurate because the "normal" level has a very wide range.

Since all the urine is collected in one container, this would not detect any of the fluctuations or variations in cortisol levels occurring during the day. Also collecting a 24-hour urine specimen is a bit onerous. However, this test is good for determining the *total cortisol*, which could be very helpful to know.

Blood measurement of cortisol is not very useful, mainly because of the wide variability of "normal" levels.

A much better test is a saliva determination of cortisol levels. Since saliva is readily produced in most people, it would be easy to get patients to take specimens at 8am, noon, 4pm and midnight. This would definitely be a more convenient method and just as accurate. However, the problem with salivary cortisol measurement is that it is a measure of *"free"* cortisol and not *"total"* cortisol. The mistake here is that practitioners have been doing salivary cortisol levels which show low "free" cortisol levels, then interpret this as "adrenal exhaustion'. The total cortisol is not low, the adrenals are not fatigued. The regulatory mechanism is what causes the "free" cortisol to be low. Since only the "free" cortisol is biologically active, this produces the "low cortisol" symptomatology.

DHEA measurement is another test that is a relatively good indicator of adrenal cortex function.

Treating "adrenal exhaustion"

It goes without saying that the stress must be reduced. There are many ways to do this, including, meditation, yoga, tai chi, mindfulness, and even regular walking and getting outside in nature are all known to have a positive effect in managing stress. It is important to build this into your routine and not simply hope it will happen. Of course, it is easier said than done.

Certain nutrients are very important to promote effective adrenal function. Supplementing vitamin C, B group vitamins, especially B_6 and pantothenic acid (B_5), zinc and magnesium can help increase adrenal function.

A good herb to start with is an adaptogen, defined as "*a nontoxic substance and especially a plant extract that is held to increase the body's ability to resist the damaging effects of stress and promote or restore normal physiological functioning.*"

(https://www.merriam-webster.com/dictionary/adaptogen accessed 25 June 2022)

Ashwagandha (Withania somnifera) is a well-known adaptogen and most "thyroid support" products will have ashwagandha as one of the ingredients.

Paul et al. (2021) showed that ashwagandha has anti-inflammatory properties as well as cortisol reducing properties. Since an elevated cortisol can have a negative effect on T4 to T3 conversion as well as a stimulatory effect on the production of rT3, it would be advantageous to reduce cortisol levels.

Such anti-inflammatory properties would be beneficial in conditions such as Hashimoto's thyroiditis, an autoimmune disease where there is always an underlying inflammation.

In a review by Mishra, Singh, and Dagenais published in 2000, the authors found that, *"Studies indicate ashwagandha possesses anti-inflammatory, antitumor, antistress, antioxidant, immunomodulatory, hemopoietic, and rejuvenating properties. It also appears to exert a positive influence on the endocrine, cardiopulmonary, and central nervous systems. The mechanisms of action for these properties are not fully understood. Toxicity studies reveal that ashwagandha appears to be a safe compound."*

Remember that hypothyroidism is, in itself, a source of stress on the body, which can put an extra burden on the adrenals.

Therefore, as stated earlier, it is not only advisable, but necessary, to treat adrenal function in the process of treating hypothyroidism.

Sharma, Basu, and Singh (2018) showed that ashwagandha is beneficial in treating subclinical hypothyroidism.

And according to Lopresti, Smith, Malva, and Kodgule (2019) ashwagandha not only works at the adrenal level but also works at the hypothalamic and thyroid level as well.

Another nutrient, not as well known, that may be worth considering is phosphatidylserine (PS). This nutrient seems to have an action at the hippocampus and hypothalamus as well as at the adrenal level. Chronic elevated cortisol from chronic stress seem to affect the cortisol receptor sensitivity. We have already discussed this. The blunting of the cortisol receptor does not switch off the ACTH release which in turn keeps stimulating the adrenals to produce cortisol. PS re-sensitises the cortisol receptor, which in turn reduces chronic elevated cortisol levels, by repairing the cortisol feedback mechanism.

PS does help to relieve stress.

Monteleone, Maj, Beinat, Natale, and Kemali (1992) showed that PS *"counteract stress-induced activation of the hypothalamo-pituitary-adrenal axis in man."* And in 2001, Benton, Donohoe, Sillance, and Nabb showed that *"the taking of 300mg PS each*

*day for a month was associated with feeling less stressed
and having a better mood.*"

In this same study, the researchers noted that PS
*"blunted the release of cortisol in response to exercise
stress"*. This could apply to any stress.

Elevated cortisol caused by stress of any type
affects sleep. PS can be used at night to help with sleep
by lowering cortisol levels.

Suggested doses are between 300 to 600 mgs.

Reducing stress and reducing cortisol goes a long
way in helping treat thyroid issues. Reducing stress is
not easy but must be dealt with, and there are ways to
reduce levels of stress.

Some suggestions are: Take up yoga, Tai Chi or
meditation; where practicable, change your job, take
regular breaks rather than waiting for a holiday once a
year, do some gentle exercise such as going for a walk.
Time out in nature, hugging a tree, is especially effective
at reducing stress levels.

Consider your diet. Improving how you eat, what
you put into your body can have a hugely positive impact
on health and well-being. Reducing, or eliminating
"junk" food is especially helpful. Reduce alcohol intake,
although some people find a little is relaxing, but restrict
your intake to a minimum. A bad diet places huge stress

on your body. Do what you can, and what is best for you. Even small changes can make a big difference.

> If "adrenal exhaustion" is suspected, that must be treated first, naturally with nutrients and/or herbs.

There are many supplement companies making a thyroid and adrenal support formulation. These usually include ashwagandha, tyrosine, iodine, selenium, and zinc. I usually recommend a supplement as above to all thyroid patients.

The good news is that "adrenal exhaustion" generally responds well to treatment and can settle down relatively quickly. Of course, this depends on the stress reduction.

For further information about adrenal issues see *You and Your Hormones, 2nd Edition.* 2020 Dr Peter Baratosy. Self-published. The book can be purchased from the author:

infoinfopeterb@gmail.com

> The thyroid can affect the adrenal glands and the adrenal glands can affect the thyroid. Both need to be treated.

Chapter 9
The thyroid/gut connection

The thyroid can affect the gut, but also the thyroid can be affected by poor gut function. So, the gut must be treated as well. Symptoms such as bloating, burping, excess flatulence, constipation, diarrhoea, etc. need to be addressed. Although many of the gut symptoms can be related to hypothyroidism, the symptoms may not necessarily be addressed totally by replacing thyroid hormone only. Extra work needs to be done to deal with the gut symptoms.

We need a good digestive system, which means adequate stomach acid and digestive enzymes to break down protein to the individual amino acids. This also assumes that there is plenty of protein in the diet. The amino acids *tyrosine* and *phenylalanine* (which can be converted to *tyrosine*) are the building blocks of T4. The absorption of these nutrients needs to be optimal.

The connection between gluten, coeliac disease and thyroid disease also needs to be explored. The connection is even more complex than we originally thought though.

The thyroid affects the gut in various ways. Hypothyroidism is associated with constipation, which is basically caused by a reduction of bowel peristalsis. Ebert (2010) maintains that all the gastrointestinal manifestations in hypothyroidism, whether in the oesophagus, stomach, or bowel, are due to reduced gut motility.

This slow bowel movement can lead to small intestine bacterial overgrowth (SIBO). Lauritano et al. (2007) showed that 54% of patients with autoimmune hypothyroidism tested positive for SIBO compared to 5% in the control group.

From this we can determine that treating the gut, treating the SIBO, needs to be part of treating hypothyroidism.

> Replacing thyroid hormone only is not enough.

Another function that slows down with hypothyroidism is bile production. Laukkarinen et al. (2003) showed that poor bile flow can lead to gall stones, as well as other gut problems.

Reduction of bile flow can also predispose to

SIBO. Bile acids promote the activation of the DIO2 enzyme. Therefore, low bile flow would interfere with thyroid hormone activation. (Watanabe et al., 2006)

The gut microbiota, the sum total of all the microbes in the gut, can affect thyroid function. Similarly, thyroid disease can affect the microbiome, SIBO, as low bile flow and a slowed transit time can all affect the microbiome (Fröhlich & Wahl, 2019).

An altered microbiome (dysbiosis) can predispose to autoimmune thyroid disease (AITD), either hypo or hyper thyroid disease, as well as other autoimmune diseases such as inflammatory bowel disease, type 1 diabetes, rheumatoid arthritis, and multiple sclerosis. The connection between AITD and dysbiosis is suggestive and more research is needed to fully confirm (Mori, Nakagawa, & Ozaki, 2012).

Yersinia enterocolitica, Helicobacter and some other gut bacteria can potentially impact on AITD. Köhling, Plummer, Marchesi, Davidge, and Ludgate (2017) discuss the association and recommend further research.

In a study by Shenkman and Bottone (1976) antibodies to *Yersinia* were found to be higher in those with thyroid disease (not just AITD but other forms of thyroid disease as well) than in normal controls. *"Antibodies were found in 24 of 36 patients with Graves' disease, five of six with autonomous adenoma, seven of seven with Hashimoto's thyroiditis, three of five with idiopathic primary hypothyroidism, four of 11 with nontoxic nodular goiter, and one of two with thyroid carcinoma."*

There is a definite relationship between Helicobacter pylori (HP) and thyroid disease, and this may be causative. Shi, Liu, Zhou, Ye, and Zhang (2013) demonstrated that cytotoxin-associated gene A (CagA) positive strains of HP are associated with autoimmune thyroid disease.

Figura et al. (2019) demonstrated that CagA strains of HP contains protein sequences similar to the thyroid and therefore can cross react with the thyroid, which may be a form of molecular mimicry.

Molecular mimicry is defined by Rojas et al. (2018) as - *"... is one of the leading mechanisms by which infectious or chemical agents may induce autoimmunity. It occurs when similarities between foreign and self-peptides favor an activation of autoreactive T or B cells by a foreign-derived antigen in a susceptible individual."*

Choi et al. in 2017 showed that anti thyroid TPO antibodies were more frequent in those with HP infection and the researchers suggested that HP may *"play a role in the development of autoimmune thyroiditis."*

Voloshyna et al. (2016) found a correlation between HP and Hashimoto's disease. They showed a higher incidence of HP in Hashimoto's patients than in controls. They also showed a reduction of TPO antibodies after successful eradication of HP.

HP can also interfere with levothyroxine absorption. A study by Bugdaci et al. (2011) shows that if a hypothyroid patient needs a large dose of levothyroxine and there is no adequate response, then HP should be considered. If found and once HP eradication occurs, the TSH, and the T3 and T4 levels will improve. One possible risk of eradicating HP is hyperthyroidism, over-replacement. This may occur because the patient is still on the large dose of levothyroxine but is now suddenly absorbing and responding to the medication.

So, the bottom line is check for HP infection with anyone with autoimmune diseases, including thyroid disease, especially if there is a history of ulcers or any gut issues or if especially large doses are needed. Since Hashimoto's does run in families, if there is no family history, this may be another clue to test for HP. Treating the HP may improve the disease.

The gut microbiota is also crucial in the metabolism of nutrients, drugs and hormones including thyroid hormone, both endogenous and exogenous (i.e., thyroid replacement). Autoimmune thyroid disease

(Hashimoto's and Graves' disease) is associated with SIBO and changes in the microbiome (Virili & Centanni, 2015).

Optimal gut function is important in thyroid disease. This is because both hypothyroidism and hyperthyroidism can affect the microbiome and the microbiome can affect the thyroid.

Zhou et al. (2014) demonstrated a significant difference in the microbiome when hyperthyroid patients were compared to healthy groups, while Su, Zhao, Li, Ma, and Wang (2020) demonstrated hypothyroidism can affect the microbiome and conversely an altered microbiome can affect thyroid function. This study was carried out on mice.

It is noteworthy that about 20% of T4 to T3 conversion occurs in the gut; this conversion depends on good gut function, including a normal microbiome (de Herder et al., 1989).

The connection between thyroid function and gut bacteria was noted by Harries as far back as 1923.

Since dysbiosis can interfere with T4 to T3 conversion, it is natural to ask if supplementing with probiotics might help with the thyroid.

In 2017, Spaggiari et al. demonstrated that there may not be a direct effect although there may be a possible interaction between probiotic supplementation and thyroid homeostasis.

While the above study was not conclusive, in general, probiotics can help the gut and a better functioning gut can possibly help the body, including the thyroid.

Hypothyroidism can cause gut inflammation which can lead to a "leaky gut syndrome" (LGS). The gut is a semi-permeable membrane that regulates what gets into the body. The contents of the gut are technically "outside" of the body, anything inside the lumen of the gut needs to be absorbed before it can be "inside" the body. So, if there is any damage to the gut lining, the regulating mechanism is damaged so that any molecule than normally isn't allowed in can get in. One of these molecules is lipopolysaccharides (LPS). LPS is a major component of gram-negative bacteria, which normally are not absorbed but if there is a LGS then LPS get into the blood stream. LPS can cause fevers, leucocytosis, platelet aggregation, thrombocytopoenia and blood clotting disorders (Rossol et al., 2011).

LPS is a very potent immune activating stimulus and plays a role in the pathogenesis of inflammatory diseases. LPS can suppress the hypothalamus-pituitary-thyroid axis and reduce TSH secretion (Kondo, Harbuz, Levy, & Lightman, 1997, Iaglova & Berezov, 2010).

All aspects of gut function can affect the thyroid, e.g., LGS, SIBO, bile acids, microbiome alterations and LPS.

Another aspect of thyroid and gut is the gluten connection. The two most common forms of thyroid disease are Hashimoto's thyroiditis (hypothyroidism) and Graves' disease (hyperthyroidism). The common factor is that both are autoimmune diseases. One thing about autoimmune diseases is that if you have one, then there is a good chance of developing others.

Freeman (2016) showed that coeliac disease (CD) has many associated autoimmune diseases including thyroid disease. CD is where there is an allergy to a protein, gluten, found in certain foods including wheat, barley, rye, and oats. Certainly, anyone with thyroid disease should be tested for thyroid antibodies and coeliac antibodies. If that person has CD, then a total gluten free (GF) diet is mandatory. If there are no coeliac antibodies, only thyroid antibodies, then a GF diet should still be suggested. I personally have seen thyroid antibodies become negative in a hypothyroid person with thyroid antibodies (Hashimoto's thyroiditis) once a GF diet was started.

So, to treat the thyroid we must also treat the gut.

Case Study

A 19-year-old lady presented with a history of hyperthyroidism. This was complicated by the fact that she was also allergic to carbimazole and PTU; the two available medications used to treat hyperthyroidism. The hyperthyroidism settled spontaneously in February 2018. She presented to me in November 2018, with recurrence of symptoms typical of hyperthyroidism, tremor, weight loss, palpitations, feeling hot, etc., despite her thyroid function test (TFT) showing only a slight TSH suppression with normal T3 and T4. (Endogenous subclinical hyperthyroidism.)

She was seeing an endocrinologist who had referred her to a surgeon with a view to thyroidectomy. She came to me for another opinion. A significant part of her history was that she was continually iron deficient. Family history included two cousins with coeliac disease (CD). I tested her coeliac antibodies, and they were extremely high, consistent with CD. She was not interested in small bowel biopsy. She stopped gluten and immediately felt better. With CD, oral iron supplements are useless because the gut damage interferes with iron absorption. I referred her for an intravenous iron infusion. Iron deficiency is a common presentation in CD.

At this early stage I cannot say if the hyperthyroidism will totally settle, or whether she will eventually need a thyroidectomy. Research shows a strong relationship between CD and autoimmune thyroid disease, mainly hypothyroidism but hyperthyroidism can occur, although less frequently (Freeman 2016). Treating the CD by totally going gluten free may resolve the hyperthyroidism and therefore prevent a thyroidectomy. A subsequent TFT was normal. Follow up continues.

Generally, it is the rule rather than the exception that gut issues are a part of any chronic condition. Common symptoms include indigestion/heartburn/ reflux, a feeling of fullness and/or feeling full hours after a meal. This would indicate hypochlorhydria, a lack of stomach acid. Also bloating, constipation, diarrhoea, excessive flatulence, abdominal pain/discomfort, as well as others.

You may be wondering, how heartburn can indicate a lack of acid. This sounds paradoxical. The gastroesophageal sphincter (GOS) and the pyloric sphincter (PyS) are controlled by acid. Acid closes the GOS. This makes sense since acid should not go up into the sensitive oesophagus as it may cause damage. The pain and burning experienced is an indication that damage is being caused.

Acid opens the PyS. When there is a normal amount of acid in the stomach, the GOS closes, and the PyS opens, and as the stomach contracts, contents go down into the duodenum. When there is a lack of acid, the GOS does not close properly, the PyS does not open properly and when the stomach contracts, the contents can go upwards. This results in reflux and heartburn. What little acid is in the stomach can cause this burning in the sensitive oesophagus.

What are the reasons for developing low stomach acid (hypochlorhydria)? There are at least three reasons, two of them have already been discussed, though not in relation to acid secretion.

1/ Stress has been shown to reduce stomach acid (Esplugues Barrachina, Beltrán, Calatayud, Whittle, & Moncada. 1996, Shiraishi, 1988).

2/ Helicobacter infection has shown to reduce stomach acid (Harris et al., 2013, Smolka & Schubert, 2017).

3/ Iatrogenic hypochlorhydria can be caused by the overuse of proton pump inhibitors (PPIs) which are drugs that inhibit acid secretion. PPIs are being overused and used for extended periods for treatment, in many cases, of simple heartburn and indigestion. (Ksiądzyna, Szeląg, & Paradowski, 2015)

Hypochlorhydria (low stomach acid) can predispose to SIBO and dysbiosis, which in turn can affect the thyroid.

One simple way of dealing with this is to *give* acid. The simplest and easiest is the use of apple cider vinegar (ACV). My recommendation is 2 tablespoons before each meal. If there is constant heartburn, the inflamed oesophagus needs to be healed first, otherwise the ACV can burn the already irritated oesophagus. This healing can be achieved by slippery elm bark (SEB).

Bloating and gurgling can be helped with the ACV, as well as probiotics, especially where there is a past history of multiple antibiotic use.

Abdominal pain can be helped with SEB – 2-3 capsules 3-4 times daily. Or it can be taken as a powder mixed with water.

The bowels need to be improved. Hypothyroidism is known to cause constipation, but just replacing thyroid hormone may not necessarily be enough.

Ask about the colour of the bowels. A light-coloured bowel action is associated with a reduction of bile production. Bile flow can be helped by dandelion root tea, 1 cup 2-3 times a day. You can see it is working by the bowel action become darker, and the constipation may ease. Increased bile flow can also act as a "soap" and help flush out the bacteria in SIBO.

Earlier I mentioned small intestinal bacterial overgrowth (SIBO). SIBO can be helped by 1/ acid supplementation and 2/ improved bile flow. The use of SEB may also be helpful to reduce gut inflammation.

Protocols include:

1/ replace stomach acid. Apple cider vinegar is a simple and easy start,

2/ encourage bile flow. Dandelion root tea is a simple way to do this,

3/ heal the gut, slippery elm bark can be very useful,

4/ supplement probiotics,

5/ improve omega 3 to omega 6 in the diet, and encourage a

6/ gluten free diet.

For full protocols see *Gut Feelings, 2nd edition* Dr Peter Baratosy. 2019. Self-published. The book can be purchased directly from the author: infoinfopeterb@gmail.com

---

The Thyroid can affect the Gut and the Gut can affect the Thyroid. Both need to be treated.

Chapter 10
The thyroid/sex hormone connection

Many with hypothyroidism are women and present in their 4th decade. Has this anything to do with menopause? Is it coincidental? Menopause is a time of hormonal imbalance, generally a relative deficiency of progesterone. Some features of menopause are similar to hypothyroidism.

Studies have shown a direct effect of oestrogen on the thyroid. Santin and Furlanetto (2011) have demonstrated that there are oestrogen receptors in the thyroid, so it follows that oestrogen does have an action on thyroid function.

The role of thyroid hormone is to convert calories to useable energy. The role of oestrogens is to store energy as fat, a totally opposite action. *Therefore, we can say that oestrogen opposes thyroid action,* possibly at the thyroid hormone receptor level.

Progesterone opposes the action of oestrogen.

Progesterone also increases the sensitivity of oestrogen receptors, but in a state of progesterone deficiency the body can secrete more oestrogen in compensation. This, and the high levels of xenoestrogenic pollution that are very common in western society leads to oestrogen dominance i.e., excess oestrogen.

Oestrogen dominance is a term used where the levels of oestrogen are out of proportion to progesterone, i.e., a *relative* oestrogen excess compared to progesterone.

This situation can arise if:

1/ the levels of oestrogen are high, and the progesterone levels are normal,

2/ the levels of oestrogen are normal, but the level of progesterone is low, or

3/ the levels of oestrogens are low, but the levels of progesterone are even lower.

Ardue et al. (2015) have shown that an imbalance of oestrogen and progesterone predisposes to the development of Hashimoto's thyroiditis, which can be associated with poly cystic ovarian syndrome (PCOS) where there is high oestrogen and low progesterone levels.

Supplementing progesterone, the natural, not the synthetic progestogens, can balance out the oestrogen dominance.

Progesterone has been shown to upregulate thyroid gene expression especially the sodium-iodide symporter (*NIS*), thyroglobulin (*TG*), and to a lesser extent the thyro-peroxidase (*TPO*). Bertoni, Brum, Hillebrand, and Furlanetto (2015) confirmed that progesterone has a direct action on thyroid function and growth.

Many of the symptoms of oestrogen dominance are akin to hypothyroidism and possibly are caused by the oestrogenic effect on thyroid function.

Santin and Furlanetto (2011) showed that excess oestrogen can block the action of thyroid hormone which leads to development of hypothyroid symptoms. This occurs at oestrogen receptor level in the thyroid gland itself.

Oestrogen has also been shown to increase thyroid binding globulin (TBG) which binds thyroid hormone, thus reducing "free" thyroid hormone. In these cases, blood tests may be normal. Women on hormone replacement or on "the pill" have been shown by Grüning, Zöphel, Wunderlich, and Franke (2007) to have a higher total T4 and total T3 and a lower "free" T3 but no change in TSH.

Taking hormones can affect the thyroid. Many women present with hypothyroidism around the menopause and a large percentage of hypothyroid patients are women. Thyroid and sex hormones do interact (Santin & Furlanetto, 2011).

Badawy, State, and Sherief (2007) state that many of the symptoms of menopause are comparable to hypothyroidism. Therefore, it would be wise to check thyroid function in menopausal women especially if they fail to respond to adequate menopausal treatment. Many women with severe menopausal symptoms should be tested and treated if thyroid hypofunction is found.

Oestrogen excess also causes the body to retain copper, thus reducing the level of zinc. This is because zinc and copper have a seesaw relationship. Zinc is an important essential nutrient needed for thyroid function. Copper is also an essential nutrient, but excess levels are known to act as an "anti-nutrient", antagonising zinc, magnesium, iron, molybdenum, manganese, vitamins B_1, C, E and folate. This can interfere with the production and utilisation of thyroid hormone, as well as a host of other hormones and biochemical processes.

It is possible that this is a reason why thyroid problems are becoming more prevalent, especially in menopausal women.

If thyroid problems do occur, they have been shown to be reversed by supplementing natural progesterone which opposes the oestrogen dominance and allows the thyroid hormones to begin working normally. Progesterone does increase free T4 levels (Sathi, Kalyan, Hitchcock, Pudek, & Prior, 2013).

Progesterone is known to increase copper excretion and therefore normalise copper (and zinc) levels.

Arafah (2001) has shown that women with hypothyroid problems, being treated with levothyroxine need to increase their dose when they start on oestrogen therapy. Steingold et al. (1991) showed that this only happens with oral hormone replacement and not with transdermal replacement.

Mazer (2004) showed that oral replacement has its effect on the liver, raising TBG which binds more T4, therefore reducing the level of "free" T4. Transdermal hormone replacement does not seem to have this problem.

The mechanism is more than likely due to the "first pass effect" where oral hormones are absorbed through the stomach and go straight to the liver. The metabolism of these hormones here puts extra stress onto the liver. Transdermal hormones bypass the liver.

Dr John R Lee (1996) was a pioneer of transdermal progesterone cream. While treating women for osteoporosis or menopausal problems with progesterone cream, he found, coincidentally that those with hypothyroidism had improved. He also noticed that women with Graves' disease and Hashimoto's thyroiditis, both auto-immune diseases, also improved. He then began to treat women, and men, with thyroid disease with progesterone cream with good results.

Graves' disease can resolve during pregnancy. Lazarus (2005) states, *"Pregnancy has marked effects on thyroid physiology and autoimmune thyroid disease tends to ameliorate through gestation due to the general immunosuppression seen in pregnancy."*

The study showed that appropriate treatment for hyperthyroidism is necessary, as just allowing the high levels of progesterone in pregnancy to deal with the hyperthyroidism may be inadequate. However, mild cases may resolve just due to the pregnancy hormones. There can be untoward effects on the pregnancy if the hyperthyroidism in not adequately controlled.

It is well known that the level of progesterone is quite high during pregnancy, and this is the reason why hyperthyroidism can reduce during pregnancy.

Oestrogen also has a role to play in promoting thyroid tumours. Women have a three times greater incidence of thyroid tumours than men. Oestrogen has been shown by Manole, Schildknecht, Gosnell, Adams, and Derwahl (2001) to stimulate the growth of benign and malignant thyroid cells. This is another instance where oestrogen dominance can play a role in thyroid disease.

The use of herbs, especially Vitex agnus castus may help hormone imbalance. This herb, the common name being the 'chaste tree berry' was known to the ancients as a treatment for many gynaecological conditions. Hippocrates (460-370 BC) wrote of this herb *"If blood flows from the womb, let the woman drink dark wine in which the leaves of the Vitex have been seeped"*.

Vitex has been shown to have a positive effect on women's issues such as PMT, breast tenderness, heavy periods, and menopausal issues.

Ahangarpour, Najim, and Farbood (2016) showed that Vitex extract has an influence on the female sex hormones although this study was done in ageing female mice.

In another study, van Die, Burger, Teede, and Bone in 2013, showed that one of the mechanisms of Vitex was on reduction of the hormone prolactin, which helps with rebalancing the other hormones, including estrogen and progesterone.

In 2017, Cerqueira, Frey, Leclerc, and Brietzke found Vitex to be safe and efficacious in treating PMT (PMS for the Americans) and premenstrual dysphoric disorder (PMDD).

Some women may need hormone replacement therapy (HRT). A better and safer hormone replacement is bio identical hormone replacement or B-HRT. This is the natural form of the hormones. Not every doctor is knowledgeable about prescribing B-HRT. There are integrative doctors who have studied the topic and are well placed to guide and assist and prescribe these products.

For years, integrative doctors have been using "natural", "bio-identical" hormone creams and have been criticized for doing so by those in orthodox medical practice. Various objections were constantly raised such as, "it doesn't work, it is dangerous, the creams do not absorb through the skin" and so on.

Things are changing.

Orthodox practitioners are now giving hormones via a patch, i.e., through the skin. They are starting to use more natural hormones such as bio-identical oestradiol, as well as micronized "real", "natural" progesterone given orally (note possible "first pass effects"). These are being called "body-identical" hormones.

The following quote from Schopenhauer (German Philosopher 1788-1860) seems appropriate at this stage.

> *"All truth passes through three stages. First, it is ridiculed. Second, it is violently opposed. Third, it is accepted as being self-evident."*

For more information about hormones see *You and Your Hormones 2nd edition.* Dr Peter Baratosy. 2020. Self-published. The book can be purchased from the author:

infoinfopeterb@gmail.com

> The thyroid can affect the sex hormones and the sex hormones can affect the thyroid. Both need to be treated.

Chapter 11
TSH "normal ranges"

One possible reason that people are told that they have "normal" blood test results is because of mistaken interpretation of the results. This could partly be due to the wide range of the "normal" TSH.

In the past, the normal ranges of TSH were very broad. A TSH at the upper end of normal may have been interpreted by some as still "normal". I personally would interpret a high "normal" TSH as being abnormal.

For example, previously, the normal range of TSH was from 0.5 to 5.5 which is a very wide range indeed.

Now the "normal" range is much narrower; 0.4 – 4.0.

What if a person had a TSH of 5.4? Technically that would be regarded as "in the normal range". But is it really?

It makes no sense that a TSH of 5.4 is normal but

a TSH of 5.6 is hypothyroid. You do not suddenly become hypothyroid when your TSH exceeds 5.5. The TSH of 5.5 is not a cut-off point, an on/off switch. I look at TSH more like a dimmer switch, a continuum. A person with a TSH of 3 is more hypothyroid than a person with a TSH of 2 and a person with a TSH of 4 is more hypothyroid than a person with a TSH of 3.

What does the "normal range" mean? I should emphasise that there is a "normal range" based on population results of the mean and two standard deviations from the mean but there is also an "optimal range".

The optimal figure for TSH is around 1-2. Note that there are people who can start to get hypothyroid type symptoms with a TSH of 3.

Early in 2001, The American Association of Clinical Endocrinologists (AACE) did a major flip-flop and revised its doctrine on how hypothyroidism should be diagnosed. In their press statement dated 18 January 2001, they said:

"Even though a TSH level between 3.0 and 5.0 uU/ml is in the normal range, it should be considered suspect since it may signal a case of evolving thyroid underactivity."

The "optimal TSH" is around 1-2.

An actual patient example will be helpful here. In many instances there may not be any previous tests when a person presents. However, there are times when previous TSH tests have been done and although their doctor told them that the result was "normal", it is the big picture that can be revealing.

```
Clinical Notes : SIGNS AND SYMPTOMS OF LOW THYROID LAST TSH
                 WAS 4.3 LOTS OF STRESS IN LIFE

THYROID FUNCTION TESTS

Date          03/08/11  30/07/13  04/02/14  09/09/14
Time F-Fast   1450      1550      1645      0820 F
Lab Id.       16495506  401023385 401307161 401543781 Units    Reference

TSH.          2.5       3.0       4.3       6.0 H    mU/L    (0.5-4.5)
```

As you can see the earlier TSH reading were "in the normal range" but you can also see that in the long-time frame, the gradual rising of the TSH possibly could indicate a developing hypothyroidism. The result on 04/02/2014 is "in the normal range" but may be suspect because; a/ it is high normal and b/ the results have been slowly increasing over time. The final reading is now in the elevated TSH range indicating hypothyroidism. There was no need to wait to commence treatment until the TSH moved into the hypothyroid range, especially if there were signs and symptoms of hypothyroidism.

Some treatment could have started earlier, e.g., diet, nutrients, and herbs.

I have seen people who told me that their doctor said to wait, to continue monitoring, and when the TSH went into the hypothyroid range, then treatment could start. Of course, conventionally, the treatment would be to start levothyroxine replacement. Conventional doctors do not know what else to do.

It is not right that a person who may have been suffering for years, must wait until their blood tests become abnormal to be treated.

When a patient comes to me and says, "My doctor told me that my TSH was 'normal'", I want to know what the actual figure was. I must admit that many new patients seeing me come prepared with a thick wad of previous test results, which can really help.

The "normal range" of TSH is changing and becoming narrower – now is 0.4 to 4.0.

This still does not answer the question of why people with a perfectly normal TSH present a clinical picture of being hypothyroid. This is the situation I call "biochemically normal but clinically hypothyroid".

The question often arises of whether it is safe to give thyroid hormone even if the blood test results are normal.

My experience shows that it is safe especially if there is regular follow up. Of course, we must correlate this with hypothyroid symptoms.

And, in response to whether you treat a person with an abnormal TFT if there are no hypothyroid symptoms? This scenario is very uncommon, but I would say "yes" with diet and supplements and not with TH replacement.

Before using thyroid replacement on anyone with the hypothyroid syndrome, a good protocol would be to use the diet, minerals and supplements as discussed earlier, as well as adrenal, gut and hormone support. If a trial of the herbs and minerals is not helping, then thyroid replacement can be commenced.

There is scientific support for this approach.

Skinner, Holmes, Ahmad, and Davies (2009) studied the responses to levothyroxine (T4), of biochemically normal but clinically hypothyroid patients. They found that T4 can be used safely to treat these patients.

The study examined 139 patients that were biochemically normal but clinically hypothyroid based on 16 recognised criteria (i.e., symptoms). They were supplemented with levothyroxine in incrementally increasing doses until the patients were clinically euthyroid. This was based on improvement of clinical features of hypothyroidism. Most patients improved, *"had favourable clinical response to thyroid replacement..."*

Chapter 12
Inflammation

As we have seen above, inflammation can influence T4 to T3 conversion.

Inflammation is a constant factor is almost every chronic disease, including the autoimmune thyroid disease, Hashimoto's thyroiditis. Therefore, treating any chronic disease involves addressing inflammation.

There are many herbs and nutrients that have anti-inflammatory activity. One herb already mentioned is ashwagandha. This herb not only has adrenal and thyroid support properties but also has anti-inflammatory and antioxidant activity. A very useful herb. Four actions for the price of one.

Another very useful herb is turmeric (Curcumin longa). Chainani-Wu (2003) and Jurenka (2009) showed that this herb has prominent anti-inflammatory action as well as an excellent safety record.

Boswellia serrate, also known as frankincense, is another potent anti-inflammatory herb. Boswellia is an ayurvedic herb that has been used in India for a very long time and is still being used as an anti-inflammatory herb. (Siddiqui, 2011)

Another nutrient that has been shown to have prominent anti-inflammatory activity is palmitoylethan-olamide (PEA).

PEA, also known as Palmidrol, is an endogenous (meaning made naturally by the body) fatty acid amide that has many actions. First discovered in 1957, many studies have shown its usefulness as a potent anti-inflammatory (Hesselink, Kopsky, & Witkamp, 2014), and analgesic which has neuro-protective, and immune system regulation activity. PEA has been described as a *cannabimimetic* but is **not** a cannabinoid. The mode of action is by enhancing the Endocannabinoid system (ECS) (Clayton, Hill, Bogoda, Subah, & Venkatesh, 2021).

Another potent anti-inflammatory is cannabidiol oil (CBD oil). This is a cannabis extract, which does not contain the psychoactive element, tetrahydrocannabinol (THC) and therefore does not get you "high". In a review by Henshaw, Dewsbury, Lim, and Steiner (2021) the anti-inflammatory action of CBD was shown to be very positive.

For more information about PEA and CBD see *CBD Oil: The Gift of Nature.* Dr Peter Baratosy. 2021 Self-published. The book can be ordered from the author:

infoinfopeterb@gmail.com.

PART 4

Chapter 13
How to treat hypothyroid syndrome – specifics

In this section I will discuss the specifics of treating the hypothyroid syndrome.

An accurate diagnosis can help e.g., Hashimoto's thyroiditis, mainly because autoimmune protocols can be added if necessary.

My approach is to concentrate on symptoms and assess progress based on elimination of those symptoms. Of course, blood tests can complement the assessment. Remember that TSH may not necessarily be a helpful measurement.

People who present to me, generally have one of the following issues:

1/ known hypothyroidism (most commonly Hashimoto's) and are on treatment with levothyroxine without or with minimal improvement of symptoms,

2/ known hypothyroidism, on treatment with levothyroxine and wants to change to desiccated thyroid,

3/ hypothyroid symptoms with normal blood tests, and being told it is *not* due to their thyroid,

4/ abnormal blood tests that are contradictory, and their regular doctors cannot make sense of it,

5/ hypothyroid symptoms and have been treated with levothyroxine and get worse,

6/ have been diagnosed with hypothyroidism but do not know what type. The most common scenario is they have Hashimoto's, but they have never been tested, or

7/ they tell me that they feel fine, there is nothing wrong, but they have a strong family history of thyroid disease, and they want to know if they can do anything to prevent it.

As any good doctor knows, the first thing to do is to take a thorough medical history. Many years ago, when I was in medical school, we were taught that in 80% of the time, you can get your diagnosis just from taking a thorough history. Another 10% of getting the diagnosis is if you do a comprehensive physical examination and finally doing various investigations can give the last 10% of getting the diagnosis.

In general practice where time is often limited to a 10–15-minute consultation, it is impossible to do all of the above, or even to do one aspect of clinical diagnosis effectively. The argument is that if you see the same person regularly then you can get the full story … eventually.

I say that is not good enough. I would like to know what is going on from the first visit.

So, in my practice, I generally see a first-time patient for a one-hour consultation and, in this time, with practice, you can take a good history, do a thorough examination and order pathology/or radiology, if needed. Then some treatment can be started, because in most cases I know what was going on. It is rare that I needed to wait for the investigation results to come back before starting some treatment. The key was thorough history taking, and physical examination. In some cases, keen observation of the patients as they came into the office was enough for me to know that they are hypothyroid.

When the patient made the appointment, I would request that they bring information about what other doctors had done, any results from previous tests and a list of anything they had been prescribed. As I talked with them, I always asked what their response was to what had been prescribed. Knowing all this makes it much easier to plan treatment for a patient.

It is not within the scope of this book to discuss how to do a full history and examination, however, below are those things specifically relevant to thyroid and associated issues.

Initial observations:

* Do they look hypothyroid? Sometimes you can tell as soon as you see a person.

* Are they overweight?

* Do they look tired?

* Do they have bags under the eyes?

* Do they have cold hands?

* Before Covid, I used to shake hands when first greeting new patients. From this you can assess if they have a cold hand. Cold hands are a symptom of hypothyroidism, or it could be just the cold weather. Or is the hand cold and clammy?

* Do they have hot dry hands?

* Do they have dry skin?

* Do they have anxiety?

* Look at their hair. Is it shiny and lustrous? Or dry and straw-like? These can all point to hypothyroidism

* Are they obese? Or thin?

* Observe how they are dressed. Are they wearing a thick jacket even in summer? If so, it may mean they are hypothyroid.

Take a good history. Concentrate on symptoms. Listen to the patient. "Doctor, I am tired and cold all the time, and putting on weight." Do not dismiss it.

Other symptoms you might notice, or they might report, are: stress, anxiety, depression, dizziness on standing, thirst and salt craving. This could indicate "adrenal exhaustion".

Are there any gut issues such as: bloating, burping, excess flatulence, constipation, diarrhoea? Other symptoms they may mention are, feeling full quickly, food sitting in pit of stomach hours after a meal, heartburn/reflux? This could mean stomach acid deficiency.

Discuss menopause symptoms with females who present, and if they are younger women, ask about any menstrual difficulties?

Check for a past history of illness, especially autoimmune disease. Have there been any thyroid issues in the past? Any operations? Also, ask if they have had, or still have any recurrent infections, (multiple antibiotic use). Do they have allergies or asthma?

Family History (FH) is important as you can learn a lot when you ask, "Is there a FH of thyroid disease, or any other diseases?"

"Why yes, my mother, grandmother, aunties, and cousins all have Hashimoto's!" I think that is significant as Hashimoto's does run in families.

Or "My sister has Graves' disease, my mother has rheumatoid arthritis, my auntie has type 1 diabetes and I have 2 cousins with coeliac disease." This indicates a strong FH of autoimmune disease, and this can also be significant. Note that in some families, the hypothyroidism (Hashimoto's) is not inherited but the tendency to autoimmunity is, which could include Hashimoto's.

It may be useful to know the occupation, e.g., if the person is a painter and decorator, consider lead or possible mercury poisoning.

Ask about hobbies. I once had a patient whose hobby was lead-lighting. She was surprised that she had some lead poisoning. Other hobbies include old house renovation which can also lead to mercury and/or lead exposure.

A dietary assessment can be very helpful. Is it a healthy, nutritious diet or a poor diet? Do they eat a lot of fish? If so, this could possibly indicate mercury. A high "junk" food diet is not healthy and certainly can put more stress onto the body.

Medications. Are they already on thyroid replacement such as levothyroxine?

If they are on supplements, what are they? Are they taking supplemental iodine or selenium?

Eyes. Is there exophthalmos? (Graves' Disease)

Eyebrows. Hertoghe's sign where there is thinning or missing of the outer third of eyebrow. This is a known sign in hypothyroidism (also known as Queen Anne's sign, so named because a portrait of her shows her eyebrow missing the outer third). The eyebrows can grow back with treatment.

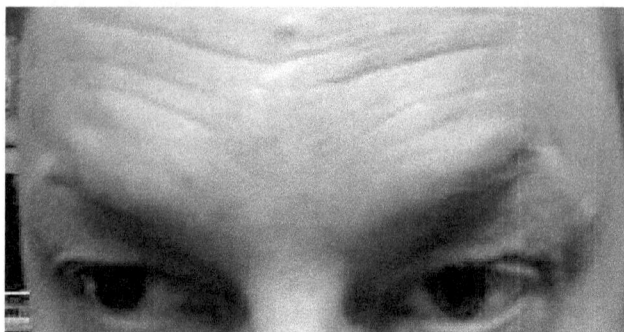

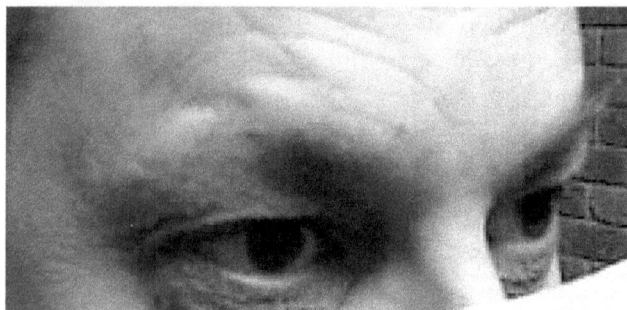

Check pupil reaction. Do they react strongly? Normally? Are they sluggish? Are the pupils unstable, i.e., do they dilate then contract then dilate then contract? This could indicate "adrenal fatigue".

An interesting sign, I named after myself is Baratosy's sign (!!) This is wearing sunglasses on their head, especially in the Tasmanian winter. This would indicate sensitivity to light which can be a sign of "adrenal fatigue". This can be explained by the muscle weakness of the circular muscle fibres in the pupil. In bright light the muscle cannot sustain the pupil constriction and the pupil dilates and this leads to the light sensitivity.

Look in the mouth. Do they have amalgams? Consider a mercury issue. If no amalgams, ask if they ever had amalgams and had them replaced with composites. Ask if they have been detoxed from mercury?

Look at the neck. Is there a goitre?

Feel pulse. Is it fast or slow? Hypothyroidism can have a slow pulse rate. Hyperthyroidism has a fast heart rate.

Blood Pressure, if low especially on standing, consider "adrenal fatigue".

Skin – dry skin?

Abdomen. Is there any bloating? This could indicate SIBO.

These are the main things to look for if considering a thyroid problem. Of course, it goes without saying that a full regular physical examination is essential as you may pick up other issues.

Chapter 14
How to start treatment

Once you have worked with the client to improve the function of the adrenals, gut, and hormones, you can start working on the thyroid. Though this can all be done concurrently.

A supplement I use regularly because it covers both thyroid and adrenal support is one which contains iodine, selenium, zinc, tyrosine and ashwagandha. This will cover both thyroid and adrenal support.

These supplements can be started before thyroid hormone (TH) is prescribed. In many cases, TH replacement may not even be necessary because the herbs and nutrients have adequately improved the situation.

If, after supplementation, and other support there is little, or no improvement, then TH can be started.

Levothyroxine is often the first choice as indicated by Skinner, Holmes, Ahmad, and Davies

(2009). While that might be a good start, I personally prefer the use of the natural desiccated thyroid (DT).

Many people come to see me specifically because they want to start DT. Unfortunately, this is not a government subsidised medication and does cost more, which makes it out of reach for some people, though many are willing to pay this extra amount because they know it works. However, as DT is made up by compounding pharmacists, some private health insurance funds may at least partially cover the cost.

Standard protocol states that we should start low and slowly increase till there is a response.

With levothyroxine, a half of a 50 microgram (mcg) levothyroxine tablet (equivalent to 25 mcg) is started daily. If after 5 - 10 days there is no response, the dose can be increased to 50 mcg. It is then increased to 75 mcg (one and a half tablets) and so on until there is a response. Once there is improvement, slow down with increasing the dose. Watch and wait and any increase may be with smaller increments. Obviously stop increasing if there are signs of hyperthyroidism, i.e., over-replacement. Temporarily stop, re-assess, and adjust dose.

As stated earlier, I prefer the natural DT.

The compounding pharmacists make the natural DT up at a dose that is determined by the doctor. i.e., the compounding pharmacist can make up capsules at any dose that is prescribed by the doctor. I generally start with a 40 mg capsule. I base this on the conversion: 50 mcg levothyroxine is equivalent to 80 mgs desiccated thyroid.

50 mcg levothyroxine is equivalent to 80 mgs desiccated thyroid.

Again, start low at 40 mgs (1 capsule daily) and slowly increase to 80 mgs (2 capsules daily) then depending on response the dose can be increased to 120 mgs (3 capsules daily). Slowly keep increasing until there is a response. Once there is a response albeit inadequate, it is advisable to increase in smaller increments (e.g., 5 – 10 mgs). Stop if there are signs of over-replacement.

How high can you go?

As mentioned above, the dose can be slowly increased until there is a response, with the limiting factor being over-replacement. Sometimes there is a fine line between an adequate dose and over-replacement.

The largest dose I have prescribed is 320 mgs. Most people are generally in the 80 to 160 mgs range.

Endocrinologists are strongly against the natural DT. They make many excuses, the main one being that each batch may be different therefore the dose needs to be changed with every new script.

I strongly refute this.

I have treated many people with DT for many years and the dose did not need to be changed with every new script. This is because the manufacturer of desiccated thyroid blends the product to produce a standardised product.

Many hypothyroid patients are extremely unhappy with their treatment. In an online survey posted on the American Thyroid Association web site, respondents were asked to rank satisfaction with their treatment and their physicians; 12,146 people completed the survey. The conclusion was that *"A subset of patients with hypothyroidism are not satisfied with their current therapy or their physicians. Higher satisfaction with both treatment and physicians is reported by those patients on DTE (Desiccated Thyroid Extract)"* (Peterson et al., 2018).

Shakir et al. (2021) showed that patients preferred DT, especially those that did not respond satisfactorily to T4. In another study, Hoang, Olsen, Mai, Clyde, and Shakir (2013) show that although there was not much difference between the T4 alone and the DT, subgroup analysis demonstrated that those not responding to T4 did better on the DT. Nearly half of the study participants preferred DT.

Patients prefer DT, possibly because they feel better. And, as it is the responsibility of the doctor to help patients feel better, it makes sense that you would provide them with the option of a therapy that can do this.

DT works, especially for those that do not respond to levothyroxine alone. And long-term DT is safe as found in a study by Tariq, Wert, Cheriyath, and Joshi (2018) Of course, doses must be monitored and adjusted as needed!

Despite the anti-DT attitude of endocrinologists, one did refer a patient to me because the patient insisted on being prescribed DT.

Chapter 15
The use of T3 in treatment

Toft (2017), and Kalra and Khandelwal (2011) suggest that in certain situations, the addition of T3 may be useful. As we have seen, T3 is the active hormone, not T4. Some individuals need a slightly higher dose of T4 to achieve euthyroidism. The downside is that the TSH may be suppressed, and this does worry the conventional doctors.

It is interesting to note what happens if, instead of increasing T4 doses, some T3 is added to the mix.

Escobar-Morreale, del Rey, Obregón, and de Escobar (1996) demonstrated that it was not possible to raise intracellular T3 levels to normal on T4 alone, at least in thyroidectomised rats. They also showed that the addition of T3 induced euthyroidism with lower doses of T4.

Bunevicius, Kazanavicius, Zalinkevicius, and Prange (1999) showed that adding T3 to T4 does improve mood and neuropsychological functioning in hypothyroid patients. Adding T3 to T4 replacement mimics the natural situation, as the thyroid does release both T3 and T4.

There have been a few studies comparing combined therapy with monotherapy.

Escobar-Morreale et al. (2005) concluded that the combination *"do not offer any objective advantage over l-thyroxine alone, yet patients prefer combination treatment."*

Why would people prefer the combination? Could it be because they felt better?

In another study, Appelhof et al. (2005) concluded *"Patients preferred combined LT4/LT3 therapy to usual LT4 therapy, but changes in mood, fatigue, well-being, and neurocognitive functions could not satisfactorily explain why the primary outcome was in favor of LT4/LT3 combination therapy. Decrease in body weight was associated with satisfaction with study medication."*

Again, why would people prefer T3 + T4 to T4 alone? Is it because they "felt better"? Isn't that the job of the doctor to make the patient feel better, to improve their quality of life?

> The doctor's job is to improve the life of their patient.

The study by Nygaard, Jensen, Kvetny, Jarløv and Faber (2009) showed that the combination of T3 and T4 was superior to T4 alone *"by evaluating several QOL (Quality of Life), depression and anxiety rating scales as well as patients own preference."*

The original treatment for hypothyroidism in the late 1800s was the use of animal thyroids, which was in essence a "combination therapy". With the development of the synthetic T4, the trend shifted to the use of these products. According to McAninch and Bianco (2019) the trend is swinging back towards the use of combined therapy. They acknowledge that the treatment of hypothyroidism should be personalised, especially since the discovery of the DIO2 SNP (Thr92AlaD2 polymorphism). Some patients do need combination therapy.

We have already acknowledged that the main TH, thyroxine (T4) is <u>not</u> the active hormone. Also note that the most usual form of thyroid replacement is with a synthetic T4, levothyroxine.

If T4 is an inactive pro-hormone, why is it given to treat hypothyroidism? I should mention here that there are numerous people with hypothyroidism who are treated with synthetic T4 and do extremely well.

However, there are those with hypothyroidism who do not respond adequately to synthetic T4, or I should say, to T4 alone. Why is T4 only used? Since the thyroid gland does release T4 and some T3, why isn't T3 also given?

Endocrinologists were very against the use of T3 but recently their attitude has changed, and some are prescribing T3 with T4, in the appropriate situation of course.

The main reason T4 only is used is the *assumption* that the T4 will be converted to T3. However, as we have seen, this assumption is not always correct.

Time for another case history.

A 45-year-old lady with Hashimoto's was initially treated with levothyroxine by the endocrinologist. Her blood test results returned to normal but clinically she was still hypothyroid symptomatically, to some degree. She did not feel well. She came to see me, and I started her on DT. She made excellent progress and in her own words *"I now feel normal again! I feel human!"*

At her follow-up appointment, it horrified the endocrinologist that she was on DT, and she was told to stop and go back onto levothyroxine. She did, but very quickly she felt awful again and came back to me. At her request the DT was re-started, and she improved almost immediately and was back to her better/normal self again. She was again followed up by the endocrinologist who was happy that she was well and the TFT was normal. She did not reveal that she was back on DT.

Chapter 16
How to treat specific situations

Below are some situations the medical practitioner may be confronted with:

The person is already taking levothyroxine and wishes to change to desiccated thyroid.

In this situation, convert the dose of levothyroxine to desiccated thyroid based on the conversion rate as mentioned above.

E.g., the person is taking 100 mcg levothyroxine. This converts to 160 mgs desiccated thyroid. I usually subtract a "fudge factor" and start a bit lower e.g., 150 mgs, then adjust the dose as needed.

The person is on levothyroxine and is still symptomatic but doesn't want to use desiccated thyroid.

In this situation add SR T3 to the levothyroxine. The starting dose would be 10 mcg SR T3, then slowly increase to 20 mcg, and then 30 mcg. If the 30 mcg is too much and the 20 is not enough, then a prescription for 25 mcg would be tried. This is all a matter of adjusting the dose in a "trial and error" fashion.

How to treat a high rT3?

Since the T4 is being converted to rT3, it would be inadvisable to supplement more T4. In this situation, SR T3 would be the prescription of choice. Here again, dosage is important. When there is a high rT3, then larger doses of SR T3 are needed. Here again, slowly increase the dose till there is a response. The highest dose I have ever prescribed is 145 mcg SR T3 daily. This is quite a high dose. If a normal person were to take this amount, they would go hyperthyroid very quickly.

A person with a high rT3 can tolerate these high doses because the rT3 has a "blocking effect" on the T3. The person with a high rT3 will start to feel "normal" at these doses.

The danger that as the rT3 levels reduce, the high T3 dose may cause a hyperthyroid state. *The person must be warned.* Should the person start to feel jittery or anxious, develop palpitations or just a fast heart rate, the dose of SR T3 needs to be reduced immediately. The reduction of rT3 levels to normal could take months, so the dose of SR T3 can also drop to a more normal level, or even be stopped.

A very important point here is that all through this process, the person must be regularly monitored either clinically, or with blood tests or with a judicious use of both. Doses must be reduced or temporarily stopped and then adjusted if there are signs of over-replacement.

There must be regular monitoring of the patient.

Over-replacement means that there is too much TH in the body. This would technically be an iatrogenic (doctor caused) hyperthyroidism.

Signs of hyperthyroidism include heat, fast heart rate or palpitations, tremor, anxiety, jitteriness, excessive weight loss, diarrhoea, (in fact many of the opposite symptoms of hypothyroidism!)

A person is NOT hypothyroid but has a strong FH and would like to prevent thyroid disease.

In this situation, blood tests should be requested for TFT, thyroid antibodies and perhaps coeliac serology if considered appropriate. Another tests that can be helpful is a spot urinary iodine.

If antibodies are present but the TFT is normal, I would suggest thyroid and adrenal support and a gluten free diet. Improve the omega 3 to omega 6 ratio in the diet. Obviously, any other condition that is found on history and examination should be treated, especially gut and hormone issues.

Chapter 17
Conclusion and summary

Treating thyroid problems is not always easy. Yes, the simple ones are straightforward, but the more complicated ones can be tricky, and most doctors do not seem to have the tools or the knowledge to manage complicated cases adequately. Hopefully after reading this book, you will have the tools and the knowledge to confidently treat any patient who presents with thyroid problems, whether straightforward or complicated.

Many doctors, even endocrinologists, treat thyroid disease to their own satisfaction, but not necessarily to the satisfaction of the patient.

If the people were treated to the point of becoming euthyroid, I would not be so busy!

All thyroid patients should be happy… but many are not.

They complain that they still have many of their original symptoms, perhaps not as severe, but the symptoms are still there. The reason is that the orthodox treatment end point is a "normal TSH". I have shown in this book that this may *not* be the end point to aim for. As doctors, our main concern must be the wellbeing of the patient. We should be aiming for removal of the symptoms. Look at the patient.

Orthodox medicine has stipulated that the biochemistry, i.e., a "normal TSH" should be the end point. There is no point treating a person to a biochemical endpoint if that person is still not clinically well. The worry is that an abnormal TSH may cause problems. Of course, an elevated TSH would indicate under-replacement BUT a "normal" TSH may not indicate adequate replacement. Some people may need a bit more TH replacement and suppress their TSH.

Remember that the TSH may not be an accurate indication of thyroid function, especially in monitoring thyroid replacement.

Doctors–listen to your patients and believe them. Do not get stuck in the present paradigm; know that a sizeable number of hypothyroid patients will not respond adequately to the sanctioned levothyroxine treatment alone. Some patients DO need added T3; do not be afraid to add it. You will be rewarded with grateful patients.

I know that doctors in general are quite conservative and, in most cases, follow strict guidelines. Unfortunately, following guidelines can make doctors lazy and prevents them from using their clinical skills. Also do not forget that all patients are different and need a personalised approach. Guidelines do not allow for flexibility. Strictly following guidelines goes against the "Art of Medicine".

This does not mean you completely ignore guidelines. At the end of this book, I have provided a flowchart. It is *not* a guideline; it is more of a logical line of thought. Use it but be open minded. Choose to use your own critical assessment skills, own knowledge, and experience rather than blindly following the guidelines … or the flowchart!

I once had a look at the official "how to treat thyroid" guidelines. I disagreed completely. None of my (complicated) patients fitted the guidelines.

Also be careful when considering guidelines. Always ask who wrote and paid for these guidelines? Pharmaceutical companies have been known to influence the writing of such documents to benefit their products.

The paradigm is slowly changing. Integrative doctors tend to use their assessment skills and work wholistically with their patients. They see patients as individuals and moderate their approach accordingly. They are using combination therapy, with either T3 and T4 or desiccated thyroid. There are now some endocrinologists who are prescribing T3.

There is a rich body of research that supports the fact that some patients do need combination therapy. Perhaps it is time that those who are developing guidelines and policies rewrote the current recommendations so that they align with what the research tells us.

There is no point to replace thyroid hormones if you under-dose. The cut-off point should be a satisfied patient without their previous hypothyroid symptoms. The cut-off point should not be determined by a biochemical result.

You need to aim for symptom removal, if not, then you are under-dosing the patient. The patient will be miserable and dissatisfied with the treatment, and with you. They will return frequently with complaints about not experiencing relief or improvement, or they will go somewhere else just to get some relief.

If you are brave enough to increase the dose to a level where the hypothyroid symptoms are relieved, you will have a happier patient.

If in increasing the dose to relieve the symptoms, the result is TSH suppression, remember that when T3 and T4 levels are normal, a suppressed TSH does not seem to produce any negative effects.

Treat the patient – not the blood test results.

Monitor the patient.

Reduce harm by monitoring the blood results, especially the level of T3. Yes, an elevated T3 can cause harm, but a normal T3, despite a suppressed TSH has not been shown to cause any issues.

In summary, remember that there is a group of hypothyroid patients that do well on T4 alone. These are the simple cases.

Conversely, there is a group of hypothyroid patients that do not get the full benefit of being treated with T4 alone. These are the people that need the addition of T3 in whatever form.

There are people who have hypothyroid symptoms but have a normal blood test. Do not dismiss them. Believe them. Remember, they have the symptoms; they are the ones suffering. Remember that what you know may not be enough. Hopefully you have learned from this book that you can treat these people with diet, minerals, herbs and with thyroid replacement.

I reiterate here that the thyroid is not an organ that exists on its own–other body systems interact with it. It is not enough to treat the thyroid in isolation. Treat all systems as mentioned earlier. These include the adrenal system, the gut and in women, the hormone system. To add to this, inflammation must also be addressed. Inflammation is everywhere where there is chronic disease.

You will find inflammation is a problem where there is pollution and where heavy metals are present. Inflammation is a particular problem where the diet is inadequate in that it is full of toxic elements and devoid of many beneficial components.

Treat the whole person–not just the thyroid.

Orthodox medicine has put fear into doctors, fear of using T3, fear of suppressing the TSH, fear of using simple, natural herbs and nutrients. The research shows that this is safe in the correct situation.

Your reward will be a happy, grateful patient.

PART 5

PART 2

Flowchart 1

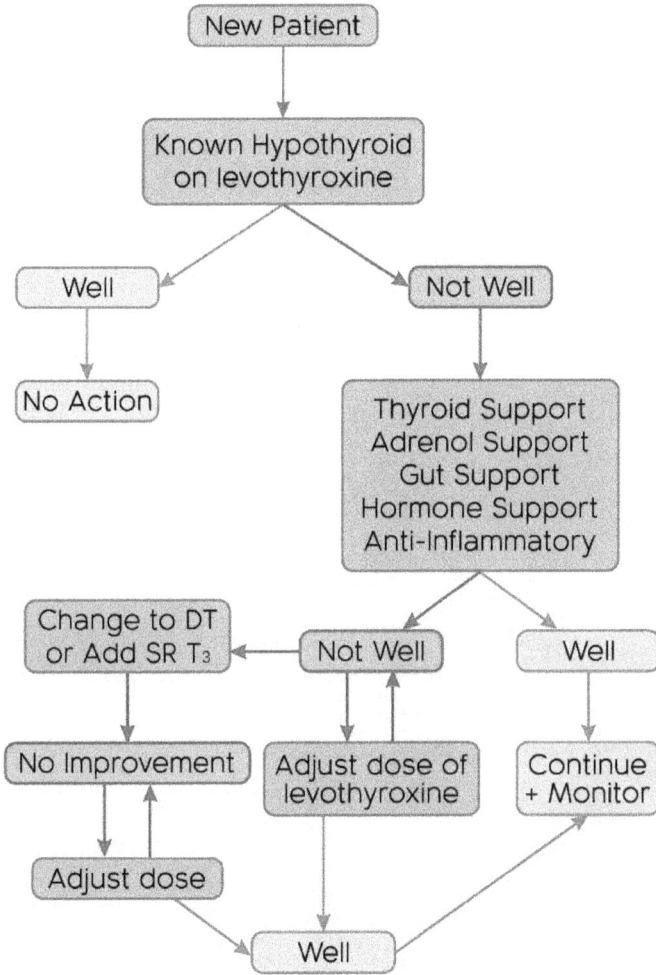

Flowchart 2

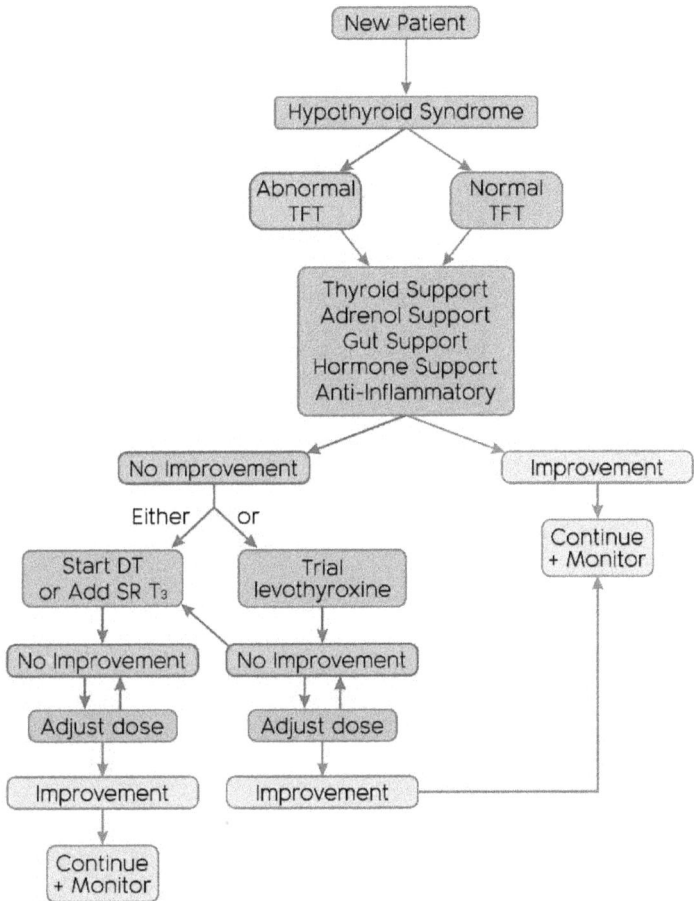

References

Abe, E., Marians, R., Yu, W., Wu, X., Ando, T., Li, Y., … Zaidi M. (2003). TSH is a negative regulator of skeletal remodeling. *Cell, 115*(2), 151-62. doi: 10.1016/s0092-8674(03)00771-2

Agocs, M., Etzel, R., Parrish, R., Paschal, D., Campagna, P., Cohen, D., … & Hesse, J. (1990). Mercury exposure from interior latex paint. *N Engl J Med, 323*(16), 1096-101. doi: 10.1056/NEJM199010183231603

Ahangarpour, A., Najimi, S. & Farbood, Y. (2016). Effects of Vitex agnus-castus fruit on sex hormones and antioxidant indices in a d-galactose-induced aging female mouse model. *J Chin Med Assoc, 79*(11), 589-596. doi: 10.1016/j.jcma.2016.05.006

Alevizaki, M., Mantzou, E., Cimponeriu, A., Alevizaki, C. & Koutras, D. (2005). TSH may not be a good marker for adequate thyroid hormone replacement therapy. *Wien Klin Wochenschr, 117*(18), 636-40. doi: 10.1007/s00508-005-0421-0

Appelhof, B., Fliers, E., Wekking, E., Schene, A., Huyser, J., Tijssen, J. … & Wiersinga, W. (2005).

Combined therapy with levothyroxine and liothyronine in two ratios, compared with levothyroxine monotherapy in primary hypothyroidism: a double-blind, randomized, controlled clinical trial. *J Clin Endocrinol Metab, 90*(5), 2666-74. doi: 10.1210/jc.2004-2111

Arafah, B. (2001). Increased need for thyroxine in women with hypothyroidism during estrogen therapy. *N Engl J Med, 344*(23), 1743-9. doi: 10.1056/NEJM200106073442302

Arduc, A., Dogan, B., Bilmez, S., Nasiroglu, N., Tuna, M., Isik, S. ... & Guler, S. (2015). High prevalence of Hashimoto's thyroiditis in patients with polycystic ovary syndrome: does the imbalance between estradiol and progesterone play a role? *Endocr Res, 40*(4), 204-10. doi: 10.3109/07435800.2015.1015730

Arthur, J., Nicol, F. & Beckett, G. (1993). Selenium deficiency, thyroid hormone metabolism, and thyroid hormone deiodinases. *Am J Clin Nutr, 57*(2 Suppl), 236S-239S. doi: 10.1093/ajcn/57.2.236S

Badawy, A., State, O. & Sherief, S. (2007). Can thyroid dysfunction explicate severe menopausal symptoms? *J Obstet Gynaecol, 27*(5), 503-5. doi: 10.1080/01443610701405812

Balazs, Z., Schweizer, R., Frey, F., Rohner-Jeanrenaud, F. & Odermatt, A. (2008). DHEA induces 11-HSD2 by acting on CCAAT/enhancer-binding proteins. *J Am Soc Nephrol*, *19*(1), 92-101. doi: 10.1681/ASN.2007030263

Baqi, L., Payer, J., Killinger, Z., Susienkova, K., Jackuliak, P., Cierny, D. & Langer, P. (2010). The level of TSH appeared favourable in maintaining bone mineral density in postmenopausal women. *Endocr Regul*, *44*(1), 9-15. doi: 10.4149/endo_2010_01_9

Bassett, J., O'Shea, P., Sriskantharajah, S., Rabier, B., Boyde, A., Howell, P., … Williams, G. (2007). Thyroid hormone excess rather than thyrotropin deficiency induces osteoporosis in hyperthyroidism. *Mol Endocrinol*, *21*(5), 1095-107. doi: 10.1210/me.2007-0033

Batrinos, M. (2006). The problem of exogenous subclinical hyperthyroidism. *Hormones (Athens)*, *5*(2), 119-25. doi: 10.14310/horm.2002.11175

Bauer, D., Nevitt, M., Ettinger, B. & Stone, K. (1997). Low thyrotropin levels are not associated with bone loss in older women: A prospective study. *J Clin Endocrinol Metab*, *82*(9), 2931-6. doi: 10.1210/jcem.82.9.4229

Bauer, M., Fairbanks, L., Berghöfer, A., Hierholzer, J., Bschor, T., Baethge, C., … Whybrow, P. (2004). Bone mineral density during maintenance treatment with supraphysiological doses of levothyroxine in affective disorders: A longitudinal study. *J Affect Disord*, *83*(2-3), 183-90. doi: 10.1016/j.jad.2004.08.011

Benton, D., Donohoe, R., Sillance, B. & Nabb, S. (2001). The influence of phosphatidylserine supplementation on mood and heart rate when faced with an acute stressor. *Nutr Neurosci, 4*(3), 169-78. doi: 10.1080/1028415x.2001. 11747360

Bernal, J., Guadaño-Ferraz, A., & Morte, B. (2015). Thyroid hormone transporters-functions and clinical implications. *Nat Rev Endocrinol, 11*(7), 406-17. doi: 10.1038/nrendo.2015.66

Bertoni, A., Brum, I., Hillebrand, A. & Furlanetto, T. (2015). Progesterone upregulates gene expression in normal human thyroid follicular cells. *Int J Endocrinol, 2015*, 864852. doi: 10.1155/2015/864852

Blum, M., Bauer, D., Collet, T., Fink, H., Cappola, A., da Costa, B., … Rodondi, N. (2015). Thyroid studies collaboration. Subclinical thyroid dysfunction and fracture risk: A meta-analysis. *JAMA, 313*(20), 2055-65. doi: 10.1001/jama.2015.5161

Bugdaci, M., Zuhur, S., Sokmen, M., Toksoy, B., Bayraktar, B. & Altuntas, Y. (2011). The role of Helicobacter pylori in patients with hypothyroidism in whom could not be achieved normal thyrotropin levels despite treatment with high doses of thyroxine. *Helicobacter, 16*(2), 124-30. doi: 10.1111/j.1523-5378.2011.00830.x

Bunevicius, R., Kazanavicius, G., Zalinkevicius, R. & Prange, A. Jr. (1999). Effects of thyroxine as compared with thyroxine plus triiodothyronine in patients with hypothyroidism. *N Engl J Med, 340*(6), 424-9. doi: 10.1056/NEJM199902113400603

Cadegiani, F. & Kater, C. (2016). Adrenal fatigue does not exist: A systematic review. *BMC Endocr Disord, 16*(1), 48. doi: 10.1186/s12902-016-0128-4

Cerqueira, R., Frey, B., Leclerc, E. & Brietzke, E. (2017). Vitex agnus castus for premenstrual syndrome and premenstrual dysphoric disorder: A systematic review. *Arch Womens Ment Health, 20*(6), 713-719. doi: 10.1007/s00737-017-0791-0

Chainani-Wu, N. (2003). Safety and anti-inflammatory activity of curcumin: A component of tumeric (Curcuma longa). *J Altern Complement Med, 9*(1), 161-8. doi: 10.1089/107555303321223035

Chan, W., Carrell, R., Zhou, A. & Read, R. (2013). How changes in affinity of corticosteroid-binding globulin modulate free cortisol concentration. *J Clin Endocrinol Metab, 98*(8), 3315-22. doi: 10.1210/jc.2012-4280

Chen, C., Chen, J., Yang, B., Liu, R., Tung, S., Chien, W. ... & Wang, P. (2004). Bone mineral density in women receiving thyroxine suppressive therapy for differentiated thyroid carcinoma. *J Formos Med Assoc,103*(6), 442-7.

Choi, Y., Kim, T., Kim, E., Jang, E., Jeon, M., Kim, W. … & Kim W. (2017). Association between thyroid autoimmunity and *Helicobacter pylori* infection. *Korean J Intern Med*, *32*(2), 309-313. doi: 10.3904/kjim.2014.369

Chopra, I., Huang, T., Beredo, A., Solomon, D., Teco, G. & Mead, J. (1985). Evidence for an inhibitor of extrathyroidal conversion of thyroxine to 3,5,3'-triiodothyronine in sera of patients with nonthyroidal illnesses. *J Clin Endocrinol Metab*, *60*(4), 666-72. doi: 10.1210/jcem-60-4-666

Clamp, A., Ladha, S., Clark, D., Grimble, R. & Lund, E. (1997). The influence of dietary lipids on the composition and membrane fluidity of rat hepatocyte plasma membrane. *Lipids*, *32*(2), 179-84. doi: 10.1007/s11745-997-0022-3

Clayton, P., Hill, M., Bogoda, N., Subah, S. & c, R. (2021). Palmitoylethanolamide: A natural Compound for health management. *Int J Mol Sci*, *22*(10), 5305. doi: 10.3390/ijms22105305

Cohen, S., Janicki-Deverts, D., Doyle, W., Miller, G., Frank, E., Rabin, B. & Turner, R. (2012). Chronic stress, glucocorticoid receptor resistance, inflammation, and disease risk. *Proc Natl Acad Sci U S A*, *109*(16), 5995-9. doi: 10.1073/pnas.1118355109 de Herder, W., Hazenberg, M., Pennock-Schröder, A., Oosterlaken, A., Rutgers, M. & Visser, T. (1989). On the enterohepatic cycle of triiodothyronine in rats; Importance of the intestinal microflora. *Life Sci*, *45*(9), 849-56. doi: 10.1016/0024-3205(89)90179-3

Ebert, E. (2010). The thyroid and the gut. *J Clin Gastroenterol*, *44*(6), 402-6. doi: 10.1097/MCG.0b013e3181d6bc3e

Elnagar, M., Abdel-Salam Dawood, A. & Abdelwahab Elshewy, E. (2018). Correlation between serum triiodothyronine level and inflammation in hemodialysis patients. *Menoufia Med J*, *31*, 402-06. doi: 10.4103/1110-2098.239722

Escobar-Morreale, H., del Rey, F., Obregón, M. & de Escobar, G. (1996). Only the combined treatment with thyroxine and triiodothyronine ensures euthyroidism in all tissues of the thyroidectomized rat. *Endocrinology*, *137*(6), 2490-502. doi: 10.1210/endo.137.6.8641203

Escobar-Morreale, H., Botella-Carretero, J., Gómez-Bueno, M., Galán, J., Barrios, V. & Sancho, J. (2005). Thyroid hormone replacement therapy in primary hypothyroidism: A randomized trial comparing L-thyroxine plus liothyronine with L-thyroxine alone. *Ann Intern Med*, *142*(6), 412-24. doi: 10.7326/0003-4819-142-6-200503150-00007

Esplugues,V., Barrachina, M., Beltrán, B., Calatayud, S., Whittle, B. & Moncada, S. (1996). Inhibition of gastric acid secretion by stress: a protective reflex mediated by cerebral nitric oxide. *Proc Natl Acad Sci U S A*, *93*(25),14839-44. doi: 10.1073/pnas.93.25.14839

Figura, N., Di Cairano, G., Moretti, E., Iacoponi, F., Santucci, A., Bernardini, G. ... & Ponzetto, A. (2019). *Helicobacter pylori* infection and autoimmune thyroid diseases: The role of virulent strains. *Antibiotics (Basel)*, *9*(1), 12. doi: 10.3390/antibiotics9010012

Freeman, H. (2016). Endocrine manifestations in celiac disease. *World J Gastroenterol*, *22*(38), 8472-8479. doi: 10.3748/wjg.v22.i38.8472

Fröhlich, E. & Wahl, R. (2019). Microbiota and thyroid interaction in health and disease. *Trends Endocrinol Metab, 30*(8), 479-490. doi: 10.1016/j.tem.2019.05.008

Fujiyama, K., Kiriyama, T., Ito, M., Kimura, H., Ashizawa, K., Tsuruta, M., ... Nagataki S. (1995). Suppressive doses of thyroxine do not accelerate age-related bone loss in late postmenopausal women. *Thyroid*, *5*(1), 13-17. doi: 10.1089/thy.1995.5.13

Garin, M., Arnold, A., Lee, J., Robbins, J. & Cappola, A. (2014). Subclinical thyroid dysfunction and hip fracture and bone mineral density in older adults: The cardiovascular health study. *J Clin Endocrinol Metab*, *99*(8), 2657-64. doi: 10.1210/jc.2014-1051

Gill R. (2014). Role of fluoride on thyroid hormone imbalance: A review. *J Adv Med Dent Sci*, *2*(2), 86-89.

Ginter, E, & Simko, V. (2016). New data on harmful effects of trans-fatty acids. *Bratisl Lek Listy*, *117*(5), 251-3. doi: 10.4149/bll_2016_048

Grant, D., McMurdo, M., Mole, P., Paterson, C. & Davies R. (1993). Suppressed TSH levels secondary to thyroxine replacement therapy are not associated with osteoporosis. *Clin Endocrinol (Oxf)*, *39*(5), 529-33. doi: 10.1111/j.1365-2265.1993.tb02404.x

Grimnes, G., Emaus, N., Joakimsen, R., Figenschau, Y. & Jorde, R. (2008). The relationship between serum TSH and bone mineral density in men and postmenopausal women: The Tromsø study. *Thyroid*, *18*(11), 1147-55. doi: 10.1089/thy.2008.0158

Grüning, T., Zöphel, K., Wunderlich, G. & Franke, W. (2007). Influence of female sex hormones on thyroid parameters determined in a thyroid screening. *Clin Lab*, *53*(9-12),547-53

Hackney, A., Feith, S., Pozos, R. & Seale, J. (1995). Effects of high altitude and cold exposure on resting thyroid hormone concentrations. *Aviat Space Environ Med*, *66*(4), 325-9.

Harries, D. (1923). The influence of intestinal bacteria upon the thyroid gland. *Br Med J, 1*(3248), 553–555. doi: 10.1136/bmj.1.3248.553

Harris, P., Serrano, C., Villagrán, A., Walker, M., Thomson, M., Duarte, I., … & Crabtree, J. (2013). Helicobacter pylori-associated hypochlorhydria in children, and development of iron deficiency. *J Clin Pathol, 66*(4),343-7. doi: 10.1136/jclinpath-2012-201243

Henshaw, F., Dewsbury, L., Lim C. & Steiner G. (2021). The effects of cannabinoids on pro- and anti-inflammatory cytokines: A systematic review of *in vivo* studies. *Cannabis Cannabinoid Res, 6*(3), 177-195. doi: 10.1089/can.2020.0105

Hesselink, J., Kopsky, D. & Witkamp, R. (2014). Palmitoylethanolamide (PEA) - 'promiscuous' anti-inflammatory and analgesic molecule at the interface between nutrition and pharma. *PharmaNutrition, 2*(1), 19-25. doi.org/10.1016/j.phanu.2013.11.127

Hoang, T., Olsen, C., Mai, V., Clyde, P. & Shakir, M. (2013). Desiccated thyroid extract compared with levothyroxine in the treatment of hypothyroidism: a randomized, double-blind, crossover study. *J Clin Endocrinol Metab, 98*(5), 1982-90. doi: 10.1210/jc.2012-4107

Holtorf, K. (2014). Thyroid hormone transport into cellular tissue. *J Restorative Medicine*, *3*(1), 53-68 doi 10.14200/jrm.2014.3.0104

Hulbert, A., Turner, N., Storlien, L. & Else, P. (2005). Dietary fats and membrane function: implications for metabolism and disease. *Biol Rev Camb Philos Soc*, *80*(1), 155-69. doi: 10.1017/s1464793104006578

Iaglova, N. & Berezov, T. (2010). Regulation of thyroid and pituitary functions by lipopolysaccharide. *Biomed Khim*, *56*(2), 179-86. Russian.

Ibarguren, M., López, D. & Escribá, P. (2014). The effect of natural and synthetic fatty acids on membrane structure, microdomain organization, cellular functions and human health. *Biochim Biophys Acta*, *1838*(6), 1518-28. doi:10.1016/j.bbamem.2013.12.021

Inoue, A., Yamamoto, N., Morisawa, Y., Uchimoto, T.,Yukioka, M. & Morisawa, S. (1989). Unesterified long-chain fatty acids inhibit thyroid hormone binding to the nuclear receptor. Solubilized receptor and the receptor in cultured cells. *Eur J Biochem*, *183*(3), 565-72. doi: 10.1111/j.1432-1033.1989.tb21085.x

Jurenka, J. (2009). Anti-inflammatory properties of curcumin, a major constituent of Curcuma longa: a review of preclinical and clinical research. *Altern Med Rev*, *14*(2), 141-53.

Kakucska, I., Qi, Y. & Lechan, R. (1995). Changes in adrenal status affect hypothalamic thyrotropin-releasing hormone gene expression in parallel with corticotropin-releasing hormone. *Endocrinology*, *136*(7), 2795-802. doi: 10.1210/endo.136.7.7789304

Kalra, S. & Khandelwal, S. (2011). Why are our hypo-thyroid patients unhappy? Is tissue hypothyroidism the answer? *Indian J Endocrinol Metab*, *15*(Suppl2), S95–S98. doi: 10.4103/2230-8210.83333

Kelly, G. (2000). Peripheral metabolism of thyroid hor-mones: A review. *Altern Med Rev*, *5*(4), 306-33.

Kis, G., Varga, A. & Lugasi, A. (2006). A comparison of chemical composition and nutritional value of organ-ically and conventionally grown plant derived foods. *Orv Hetil*, *147*(43), 2081-90.

Klein, I. & Danzi, S. (2007). Thyroid disease and the heart. *Circulation*, *116*(15), 1725-35. doi: 10.1161/CIRCULATIONAHA.106.678326

Köhling, H., Plummer, S., Marchesi, J., Davidge, K. & Ludgate, M. (2017). The microbiota and autoimmunity: Their role in thyroid autoimmune diseases. *Clin Immu-nol*, *183*, 63-74. doi: 10.1016/j.clim.2017.07.001

Kondo, K., Harbuz, M., Levy, A. & Lightman, L. (1997). Inhibition of the hypothalamic-pituitary-thyroid axis in response to lipopolysaccharide is independent of changes in circulating corticosteroids. *Neuroimmuno-modulation*, *4*(4), 188-94. doi: 10.1159/000097337

Koulouri, O., Moran, C., Halsall, D., Chatterjee, K. & Gurnell, M. (2013). Pitfalls in the measurement and interpretation of thyroid function tests. *Best Pract Res Clin Endocrinol Metab*, *7*(6), 745-62. doi: 10.1016/j.beem.2013.10.003

Książdzyna, D., Szeląg, A. & Paradowski, L. (2015). Overuse of proton pump inhibitors. *Pol Arch Med Wewn*, *125*(4), 289-98. doi: 10.20452/pamw.2790

Kurutas, E. (2016). The importance of antioxidants which play the role in cellular response against oxidative/nitrosative stress: Current state. *Nutr J*, *5*(1), 71. doi: 10.1186/s12937-016-0186-5

Laukkarinen, J., Sand, J., Saaristo, R., Salmi, J., Turjanmaa, V., Vehkalahti, P. & Nordback, I. (2003) Is bile flow reduced in patients with hypothyroidism? *Surgery*, 133(3), 288-93. doi: 10.1067/msy.2003.77

Lauritano, E., Bilotta, A,, Gabrielli, M., Scarpellini, E., Lupascu, A., Laginestra, A. … & Gasbarrini A. (2007). Association between hypothyroidism and small intestinal bacterial overgrowth. *J Clin Endocrinol Metab*, *92*(11), 4180-4. doi: 10.1210/jc.2007-0606

Lazarus, J. (2005). Hyperthyroidism during pregnancy: Etiology, diagnosis and management. *Womens Health (Lond)*, *1*(1), 97-104. doi: 10.2217/17455057.1.1.97

Lee, John R. (1996). *What Your Doctor May Not Tell You About Menopause* New York, NY: Little Brown.

Lee, M., Park, J., Bae, K., Jee, Y., Ko, A., Han, Y., ... Kang SJ. (2014). Bone mineral density and bone turnover markers in patients on long-term suppressive levothyroxine therapy for differentiated thyroid cancer. *Ann Surg Treat Res*, *86*(2), 55-60. doi: 10.4174/astr.2014.86.2.55

Lee, S & Farwell, A (2016). Euthyroid sick syndrome. *Compr Physiol*, *6*(2),1071-80. doi: 10.1002/cphy.c150017.

Ling, C., Sun, Q., Khang, J., Felipa Lastarria, M., Strong, J., Stolze, B. ... & Soldin, S. (2018). Does TSH reliably detect hypothyroid patients? *Ann Thyroid Res*. *4*(1), 122-125.

Lopresti, A., Smith, S., Malvi, H. & Kodgule, R. (2019). An investigation into the stress-relieving and pharmacological actions of an ashwagandha (Withania somnifera) extract: A randomized, double-blind, placebo-controlled study. *Medicine (Baltimore)*, *98*(37), e17186. doi:10.1097/MD.0000000000017186

Lyons, G., Judson, G., Ortiz-Monasterio, I., Genc, Y., Stangoulis, J. & Graham, R. (2005). Selenium in Australia: Selenium status and biofortification of wheat for better health. *J Trace Elem Med Biol*, *19*(1), 75-82. doi: 10.1016/j.jtemb.2005.04.005

Mancini, A., Di Segni, C., Raimondo, S., Olivieri, G., Silvestrini, A., Meucci, E. & Currò, D. (2016). Thyroid hormones, oxidative stress, and inflammation. *Mediators Inflamm*, *2016*, 6757154. doi: 10.1155/2016/6757154

Maninger, N., Capitanio, J., Mason, W., Ruys, J. & Mendoza, S. (2010). Acute and chronic stress increase DHEAS concentrations in rhesus monkeys. *Psychoneuroendocrinology*, *35*(7), 1055-62. doi: 10.1016/j.psyneuen.2010.01.006

Manole, D., Schildknecht, B., Gosnell, B., Adams, E, & Derwahl, M. (2001). Estrogen promotes growth of human thyroid tumor cells by different molecular mechanisms. *J Clin Endocrinol Metab*, *86*(3), 1072-7. doi: 10.1210/jcem.86.3.7283

Marcocci, C., Golia, F., Bruno-Bossio, G., Vignali, E. & Pinchera, A. (1994). Carefully monitored levothyroxine suppressive therapy is not associated with bone loss in premenopausal women. *J Clin Endocrinol Metab*, *78*(4), 818-23. doi: 10.1210/jcem.78.4.8157704

Mattos, G., Heinzmann, J., Norkowski, S., Helbling, J., Minni, A., Moisan, M. & Touma, C. (2013). Corticosteroid-binding globulin contributes to the neuroendocrine phenotype of mice selected for extremes in stress reactivity. *J Endocrinol*, *219*(3), 217-29. doi: 10.1530/JOE-13-0255

Maydych, V., Claus, M., Watzl, C. & Kleinsorge, T. (2018). Attention to Emotional Information Is Associated With Cytokine Responses to Psychological Stress. *Front Neurosci*, *12*, 687. doi: 10.3389/fnins.2018.00687

Mazer, N. (2004). Interaction of estrogen therapy and thyroid hormone replacement in postmenopausal women. *Thyroid*, *14 Suppl 1*, S27-34. doi: 10.1089/105072504323024561

Mazziotti, G., Sorvillo, F., Piscopo, M., Cioffi, M., Pilla, P., Biondi, B. … & Carella, C. (2005). Recombinant human TSH modulates in vivo C-telopeptides of type-1 collagen and bone alkaline phosphatase, but not osteoprotegerin production in postmenopausal women monitored for differentiated thyroid carcinoma. *J Bone Miner Res*, *20*(3), 480-6. doi: 10.1359/JBMR.041126

McAninch, E. & Bianco, A. (2019). The swinging pendulum in treatment for hypothyroidism: From (and toward?) combination therapy. *Front Endocrinol (Lausanne)*, *10*, 446. doi: 10.3389/fendo.2019.00446

McCormack, P., Reed, H., Thomas, J. & Malik, M. (1996). Increase in rT3 serum levels observed during extended Alaskan field operations of Naval personnel. *Alaska Med, 38*(3), 89-97

McDermott, M. (2012). Does combination T4 and T3 therapy make sense? *Endocr Pract, 18*(5), 750-7. doi: 10.4158/EP12076.RA

Merkulov, V., Merkulova, T. & Bondar, N. (2017). Mechanisms of brain glucocorticoid resistance in stress-induced psychopathologies. *Biochemistry (Mosc), 82*(3), 351-365. doi: 10.1134/S0006297917030142

Midgley, J., Toft, A., Larisch, R., Dietrich, J. & Hoermann, R. (2019). Time for a reassessment of the treatment of hypothyroidism. *BMC Endocr Disord, 19*, 37. doi.org/10.1186/s12902-019-0365-4

Mishra, L., Singh, B. & Dagenais, S. (2000). Scientific basis for the therapeutic use of Withania somnifera (ashwagandha): A review. *Altern Med Rev, 5*(4), 334-46.

Monteleone, P., Maj, M., Beinat, L., Natale, M. & Kemali, D. (1992). Blunting by chronic phosphatidylserine administration of the stress-induced activation of the hypothalamo-pituitary-adrenal axis in healthy men. Eur *J Clin Pharmacol, 42*(4), 385-8. doi: 10.1007/BF00280123

Morgan 3rd, C., Southwick, S., Hazlett, G., Rasmusson, A., Hoyt, G., Zimolo, Z. & Charney, D. (2004). Relationships among plasma dehydroepiandrosterone sulfate and cortisol levels, symptoms of dissociation, and objective performance in humans exposed to acute stress. *Arch Gen Psychiatry*, *61*(8), 819-25. doi: 10.1001/archpsyc.61.8.819

Mori, K., Nakagawa, Y. & Ozaki, H. (2012). Does the gut microbiota trigger Hashimoto's thyroiditis? *Discov Med*, *14*(78), 321-6.

Mori, K., Yoshida, K., Tani, J., Hoshikawa, S., Ito, S. & Watanabe, C. (2006). Methylmercury inhibits type II 5'-deiodinase activity in NB41A3 neuroblastoma cells. *Toxicol Lett*, *161*(2), 96-101. doi: 10.1016/j.toxlet.2005.08.001

Nygaard, B., Jensen, E., Kvetny, J., Jarløv, A. & Faber, J. (2009). Effect of combination therapy with thyroxine (T4) and 3,5,3'-triiodothyronine versus T4 monotherapy in patients with hypothyroidism, a double-blind, randomised cross-over study. *Eur J Endocrinol*, *161*(6), 895-902. doi: 10.1530/EJE-09-0542

Okamoto, R. & Leibfritz, D. (1997). Adverse effects of reverse triiodothyronine on cellular metabolism as assessed by 1H and 31P NMR spectroscopy. *Res Exp Med (Berl)*, *197*(4),211-7. doi: 10.1007/s004330050070

Panicker, V., Saravanan, P., Vaidya, B., Evans, J., Hattersley, A., Frayling, T. & Dayan, C. (2009). Common variation in the DIO2 gene predicts baseline psychological well-being and response to combination thyroxine plus triiodothyronine therapy in hypothyroid patients. *J Clin Endocrinol Metab*, *94*(5), 1623-9. doi: 10.1210/jc.2008-1301

Papadimitriou, A., Papadimitriou, D., Papadopoulou, A., Nicolaidou, P. & Fretzayas, A. (2007). Low TSH levels are not associated with osteoporosis in childhood. *Eur J Endocrinol*, *157*(2), 221-3. doi: 10.1530/EJE-07-0247

Paul, S., Chakraborty, S., Anand, U., Dey, S., Nandy, S., Ghorai, M. ... & Dey, A. (2021). Withania somnifera (L.) Dunal (Ashwagandha): A comprehensive review on ethnopharmacology, pharmacotherapeutics, biomedicinal and toxicological aspects. *Biomed Pharmacother*, *143*, 112175. doi: 10.1016/j.biopha.2021.112175

Peckham, S., Lowery, D. & Spencer, S. (2015). Are fluoride levels in drinking water associated with hypothyroidism prevalence in England? A large observational study of GP practice data and fluoride levels in drinking water. *J Epidemiol Community Health*, *69*(7), 619-24. doi: 10.1136/jech-2014-204971

Peterson, S., Cappola, A., Castro, M., Dayan, C., Farwell, A., Hennessey, J. ... & Bianco, A. (2018). An online survey of hypothyroid patients demonstrates prominent dissatisfaction. *Thyroid*, *28*(6), 707-721. doi: 10.1089/thy.2017.0681

Poomthavorn, P., Mahachoklertwattana, P., Ongphiphadhanakul, B., Preeyasombat, C. & Rajatanavin, R. (2005). Exogenous subclinical hyperthyroidism during adolescence: effect on peak bone mass. *J Pediatr Endocrinol Metab*, *18*(5), 463-9. doi: 10.1515/jpem.2005.18.5.463

Pranjić, N., Nuhbegović, S., Brekalo-Lazarević, S. & Kurtić, A. (2012). Is adrenal exhaustion synonym of syndrome burnout at workplace? *Coll Antropol*, *36*(3), 911-9.

Prigent, H., Maxime, V. & Annane, D. (2003). Clinical review: Corticotherapy in sepsis. *Crit Care*, *8*(2), 122-9. doi: 10.1186/cc2374

Pritchard, J. (1979). Toxic substances and cell membrane function. *Fed Proc*, *38*(8), 2220-5.

Quan, M., Pasieka, J. & Rorstad, O. (2002). Bone mineral density in well-differentiated thyroid cancer patients treated with suppressive thyroxine: a systematic overview of the literature. *J Surg Oncol*, *79*(1), 62-9; discussion 69-70. doi: 10.1002/jso.10043

Rezaei, M., Javadmoosavi, S., Mansouri, B., Azadi, N., Mehrpour, O. & Nakhaee, S. (2019). Thyroid dyfunction: How concentration of toxic and essential elements contributes to risk of hypothyroidism, hyperthyroidism, and thyroid cancer. *Environ Sci Pollut Res Int*, *26*(35), 35787-35796. doi: 10.1007/s11356-019-06632-7

Rojas, M., Restrepo-Jiménez, P., Monsalve, D., Pacheco, Y., Acosta-Ampudia, Y., Ramírez-Santana, C. ... & Anaya, J. (2018). Molecular mimicry and autoimmunity. *J Autoimmun*, *95*, 100-123. doi: 10.1016/j.jaut.2018.10.012

Rossol, M., Heine, H., Meusch, U., Quandt, D., Klein, C., Sweet, M. & Hauschildt, S. (2011). LPS-induced cytokine production in human monocytes and macrophages. *Crit Rev Immunol*, *31*(5), 379-446. doi: 10.1615/critrevimmunol.v31.i5.20

Rubello, D., Sonino, N., Casara, D., Girelli, M., Busnardo, G. & Boscaro, M. (1992). Acute and chronic effects of high glucocorticoid levels on hypothalamic-pituitary-thyroid axis in man. *J Endocrinol Invest*, *15*(6), 437-41. doi: 10.1007/BF03348767

Samuels, M. & McDaniel, P. (1997). Thyrotropin levels during hydrocortisone infusions that mimic fasting-induced cortisol elevations: a clinical research center study. *J Clin Endocrinol Metab*, *82*(11), 3700-4. doi: 10.1210/jcem.82.11.4376

Santin, A. & Furlanetto, T. (2011). Role of estrogen in thyroid function and growth regulation. *J Thyroid Res, 2011*, 875125. doi: 10.4061/2011/875125

Sathi, P., Kalyan, S., Hitchcock, C., Pudek, M. & Prior, J. (2013). Progesterone therapy increases free thyroxine levels-data from a randomized placebo-controlled 12-week hot flush trial. *Clin Endocrinol (Oxf), 79*(2), 282-7. doi: 10.1111/cen.12128

Schweizer, U. & Köhrle, J. (2013). Function of thyroid hormone transporters in the central nervous system. *Biochim Biophys Acta, 1830*(7), v3965-73. doi: 10.1016/j.bbagen.2012.07.015

Shakir, M., Brooks, D., McAninch, E., Fonseca, T., Mai, V., Bianco, A. & Hoang, T. (2021). Comparative Effectiveness of Levothyroxine, Desiccated Thyroid Extract, and Levothyroxine+Liothyronine in Hypothyroidism. *J Clin Endocrinol Metab, 106*(11), e4400-e4413. doi: 10.1210/clinem/dgab478

Shapiro, L., Sievert, R., Ong, L., Ocampo, E., Chance, R., Lee, M. … & Surks, M. (1997). Minimal cardiac effects in asymptomatic athyreotic patients chronically treated with thyrotropin-suppressive doses of L-thyroxine. *J Clin Endocrinol Metab, 82*(8), 2592-5. doi: 10.1210/jcem.82.8.4155

Sharma, A., Basu, I. & Singh, S. (2018). Efficacy and Safety of Ashwagandha Root Extract in Subclinical

Hypothyroid Patients: A Double-Blind, Randomized Placebo-Controlled Trial. *J Altern Complement Med*, *24*(3), 243-248. doi: 10.1089/acm.2017.0183

Shashi, S. & Singla, S. (2013). Clinical and Biochemical Profile of Deiodinase Enzymes and Thyroid Function Hormones in Patients of Fluorosis. *Aust J Basic Appl Sci*, *7*(4), 100-107.

Sheikh, S., Parikh, T., Kushchayeva, Y., Stolze, B., Masika, L., Ozarda, Y. … & Soldin, S. (2018). TSH Should not be used as a single marker of thyroid function. *Annals Thyroid Res*, *4*(2), 151-154.

Shenkman, L. & Bottone, E. (1976). Antibodies to Yersinia enterocolitica in thyroid disease. *Ann Intern Med*, *85*(6), 735-9. doi: 10.7326/0003-4819-85-6-735

Shi, W., Liu, W., Zhou, X., Ye, F. & Zhang, G. (2013). Associations of Helicobacter pylori infection and cytotoxin-associated gene A status with autoimmune thyroid diseases: a meta-analysis. *Thyroid*, *23*(10), 1294-300. doi: 10.1089/thy.2012.0630

Shiraishi, T. (1988). Hypothalamic control of gastric acid secretion. *Brain Res Bull, 20*(6),791-7. doi: 10.1016/0361-9230(88)90093-7

Siddiqui M. (2011). Boswellia serrata, a potential anti-inflammatory agent: an overview. *Indian J Pharm Sci, 73*(3), 255-61. doi: 10.4103/0250-474X.93507

Singh, N., Verma, K., Verma, P., Sidhu, G., & Sachdeva, S. (2014). A comparative study of fluoride ingestion levels, serum thyroid hormone & TSH level derangements, dental fluorosis status among school children from endemic and non-endemic fluorosis areas. *SpringerPlus, 3,*7. Doi: c10.1186/2193-1801-3-7

Skinner, G., Holmes, D., Ahmad, A. & Davies, J. (2009). Clinical Response to Thyroxine Sodium in Clinically Hypothyroid but Biochemically Euthyroid Patients. *Journal of Nutritional & Environmental Medicine, 10*(2), 115-124. doi:10.1080/13590840050043530

Smolka, A, & Schubert, M. (2017). Helicobacter pylori-Induced Changes in Gastric Acid Secretion and Upper Gastrointestinal Disease. *Curr Top Microbiol Immunol, 400,* 227-252. doi: 10.1007/978-3-319-50520-6_10

Spaggiari, G., Brigante, G., De Vincentis, S., Cattini, U., Roli, L., De Santis, M., … Santi, D. (2017). Probiotics Ingestion Does Not Directly Affect Thyroid Hormonal Parameters in Hypothyroid Patients on Levothyroxine Treatment. *Front Endocrinol (Lausanne), 8,* 316. doi: 10.3389/fendo.2017.00316

Spector, A. & Yorek, M. (1985). Membrane lipid composition and cellular function. *J Lipid Res, 26*(9), 1015-35.

Spiller, H. (2018). Rethinking mercury: the role of selenium in the pathophysiology of mercury toxicity. *Clin Toxicol (Phila)*, *56*(5), 313-326. doi: 10.1080/15563650.2017.1400555

St J O'Reilly, D. (2010). Thyroid hormone replacement: an iatrogenic problem. *Int J Clin Pract, 64*(7), 991-4. doi: 10.1111/j.1742-1241.2009.02317.x

Steingold, K., Matt, D., DeZiegler, D., Sealey, J., Fratkin, M. & Reznikov, S. (1991). Comparison of transdermal to oral estradiol administration on hormonal and hepatic parameters in women with premature ovarian failure. *J Clin Endocrinol Metab*, *73*(2), 275-80. doi: 10.1210/jcem-73-2-275

Su, X., Zhao, Y., Li, Y., Ma, S. & Wang, Z. (2020). Gut dysbiosis is associated with primary hypothyroidism with interaction on gut-thyroid axis. *Clin Sci (Lond)*, *134*(12), 1521-1535. doi: 10.1042/CS20200475

Svare, A., Nilsen, T., Bjøro, T., Forsmo, S., Schei, B. & Langhammer, A. (2009). Hyperthyroid levels of TSH correlate with low bone mineral density: the HUNT 2 study. *Eur J Endocrinol*, *161*(5), 779-86. doi: 10.1530/EJE-09-0139

Swathi, K., Haseena, S. & Saheb Shaik, H. (2014). Effect of TSH Suppression Therapy on Bone Density in Hypothyroidism. *J Pharm Sci Res*, *6*(2), 104-111.

Tabachnick, M. & Korcek, L. (1986). Effect of long-chain fatty acids on the binding of thyroxine and triiodothyronine to human thyroxine-binding globulin. *Biochim Biophys Acta*, *881*(2), 292-6. doi: 10.1016/0304-4165(86)90016-4

Tariq, A., Wert, Y., Cheriyath, P. & Joshi, R. (2018). Effects of Long-Term Combination LT4 and LT3 Therapy for Improving Hypothyroidism and Overall Quality of Life. *South Med J*, *111*(6), 363-369. doi: 10.14423/SMJ.0000000000000823

Toft, A. (2017). Thyroid hormone replacement - a counterblast to guidelines. *J R Coll Physicians Edinb*, *47*(4), 307-309. doi: 10.4997/JRCPE.2017.401

Toft, A. & Boon, N. (2000). Thyroid disease and the heart. *Heart*, *84*(4), 455-60. doi: 10.1136/heart.84.4.455

van Die, M., Burger, H., Teede, H. & Bone. K. (2013). Vitex agnus-castus extracts for female reproductive disorders: a systematic review of clinical trials. *Planta Med*, *79*(7), 562-75. doi: 10.1055/s-0032-1327831

Verhoog, N., Allie-Reid, F., Vanden Berghe, W., Smith, C., Haegeman, G. ... & Louw, A. (2014). Inhibition of corticosteroid-binding globulin gene expression by glucocorticoids involves C/EBPβ. *PLoS One*, *9*(10), e110702. doi: 10.1371/journal.pone.0110702

Virili, C. & Centanni, M. (2015). Does microbiota composition affect thyroid homeostasis? *Endocrine*, *49*(3), 583-7. doi: 10.1007/s12020-014-0509-2

Visser, J. (2013). Thyroid hormone transporters and resistance. *Endocr Dev*, *24*, 1-10. doi: 10.1159/000343695

Voloshyna, I., Krivenko, V., Voloshyn, M., Deynega, V. & Ponomarenko, V. (2016). Autoimmune thyroid disease related to Helicobacter pylori contamination. *Endocrine Abstracts*, *41*, GP213. doi: 10.1530/endo-abs.41.GP213

Waring, A., Harrison, S., Fink, H., Samuels, M., Cawthon, P, Zmuda, J., … & Bauer, D. (2013). Osteoporotic fractures in men (MrOS) Study. A prospective study of thyroid function, bone loss, and fractures in older men: The MrOS study. *J Bone Miner Res*, *28*(3), 472-9. doi: 10.1002/jbmr.1774

Watanabe, M., Houten, S., Mataki, C., Christoffolete, M., Kim, B., Sato, H. … & Auwerx, J. (2006). Bile acids induce energy expenditure by promoting intracellular thyroid hormone activation. *Nature*, *439*(7075), 484-9. doi: 10.1038/nature04330

Wiersinga, W., Chopra, I. & Teco, G. (1988). Inhibition of nuclear T3 binding by fatty acids. *Metabolism*, *37*(10), 996-1002. doi: 10.1016/0026-0495(88)90159-x

Wu, H., Xia, Y. & Chen, X. (1995). [Selenium deficiency and thyroid hormone metabolism and function.] [Article in Chinese] *Sheng Li Ke Xue Jin Zhan*, *26*(1), 12-6.

Yamamoto, N., Li, Q., Mita, S., Morisawa, S. & Inoue, A. (2001). Inhibition of thyroid hormone binding to the nuclear receptor by mobilization of free fatty acids. *Horm Metab Res*, *33*(3), 131-7. doi: 10.1055/s-2001-14939

Ye, B., Kim, B., Jeon, M., Kim, S., Kim, H., Jang, T. ... & Hong, Y. (2016). Evaluation of mercury exposure level, clinical diagnosis and treatment for mercury intoxication. *Ann Occup Environ Med*, *28*, 5. doi: 10.1186/s40557-015-0086-8

Yu, J. & Koenig, R. (2000). Regulation of hepatocyte thyroxine 5'-deiodinase by T3 and nuclear receptor co-activators as a model of the sick euthyroid syndrome. *J Biol Chem*, *275*(49), 38296-301. doi: 10.1074/jbc.M004866200

Zhang, P., Xi, H. & Yan, R. (2018). Effects of thyrotropin suppression on lumbar bone mineral density in postmenopausal women with differentiated thyroid carcinoma. *Onco Targets Ther*, *11*, 6687-6692. doi: 10.2147/OTT.S171282

Zhou, L., Li, X., Ahmed, A., Wu, D., Liu, L., Qiu, J. ... & Xin, Y. (2014). Gut microbe analysis between hyperthyroid and healthy individuals. *Curr Microbiol*, *69*(5), 675-80. doi: 10.1007/s00284-014-0640-6